Anonymus

Hebe

The art of preserving beauty and correcting deformity

Anonymus

Hebe

The art of preserving beauty and correcting deformity

ISBN/EAN: 9783742816832

Manufactured in Europe, USA, Canada, Australia, Japa

Cover: Foto ©Lupo / pixelio.de

Manufactured and distributed by brebook publishing software
(www.brebook.com)

Anonymus

Hebe

H E B E;

OR,

THE ART OF

PRESERVING BEAUTY,

AND

CORRECTING DEFORMITY;

BEING

A COMPLETE TREATISE

ON THE

Various Defects of the human Body, with the moſt approved Methods of Prevention and Cure; and the Preſervation of Health and Beauty in general.

INCLUDING AN EXTENSIVE COLLECTION OF SIMPLE YET EFFICACIOUS.

COSMETIC AND MEDICAL RECIPES,

FOR

Eſſences, Pomatums, and Waſhes for the Complexion; Liniments for thickening, ſtrengthening, and preſerving the Hair, and changing its Colour; Dentrifices for cleanſing and whitening the Teeth, preſerving the Gums; ſweetening the Breath; and curing the Tooth-ach: Remedies for Pimples, Freckles, Warts, Corns, Chilblains, and every blemiſh injurious to Beauty.

***

LONDON:

Printed for J. WALKER, No. 44, in PATER-NOSTER-ROW.

MDCCLXXXVI.

PREFACE.

THE defign of the following work is to exhibit a rational method of preventing and correcting the natural or accidental deformities and blemifhes of the human body, and of improving and heightening natural beauty.—Such a work, founded upon juft principles, will, it is hoped, prove of general utility.

Phyficians feem hitherto to have confidered whatever relates to *Cofmetics*, or the prefervation of beauty, as a fubject beneath the dignity of their pen : hence it has been confined chiefly to mifcellaneous collections of *Recipes*, often dangerous, often abfurd in their compofition, and generally ufelefs from the want of difcriminating their application ; as we fhall prefently fhew.

It is not from the *novelty* of the fubject, therefore, but from the comprehenfive and

A   connect

connect manner of treating it, that the writer hopes for approbation. Such is the natural love of mankind for the embellishment of their perfons, that above two thoufand years ago they had begun to cultivate this art. — *Heraclides*, of *Tarentum*, dedicated a treatife on Cofmetics to *Antiochis*, with whom he had fallen in love. *Mofhion* and *Mercurialis* wrote on the blemifhes of the complexion. *Artemifia*, queen of *Caria*, (who, for affection to her hufband, will ever remain the admiration of future ages) very much cultivated this fubject. *Arpafia*, the beautiful Perfian lady, who captivated the hearts of all the neighbouring monarchs, has left to the fair fex a collection of precepts for the prefervation of health and beauty, of which we find feveral fragments in the works of *Ætius*. We have likewife a book on the fame fubject, entitled, *Cleopatræ Græcorum Libri*, attributed to the famous Egyptian queen, of amorous memory, from whom fucceeding writers have borrowed

rowed many of their compofitions. Thus, though we have not the merit of being the firft who have written upon the fubjeft, yet there is a circumftance in our favour that is often decifive of an author's fuccefs,—that of being the lateft.

It is certainly not only excufeable, but highly commendable to pay attention to perfonal accomplifhments, and the gracefulnefs of the body, while fuch attention is confined within certain bounds, the extent of which reafon will dictate, though cuftom may greatly influence. We are born for each other; and therefore it is a duty we owe to fociety, as well as ourfelves, to endeavour to be mutually agreeable; and to prevent or correct every thing fhocking and difguftful. Indeed, a regard to perfonal decency fhould never be neglected, even in a ftate of perfect folitude : it would be an infult to ourfelves, and derogatory to the refpect we owe to our Creator. Perfonal negligence not only implies an infufferable indolence, but an indifference whether we pleafe or not. It often, too, betrays an infolence and affectation, arifing from a prefumption of being fure to pleafe, without having recourfe to the means which others are obliged to ufe.—Such are the principles upon which the following treatife is founded.

The FIRST BOOK is an introduction to the others, and contains a general defcription of the external parts of the human body; examining, indeed, thofe parts only which are moft liable to deformity by nature or accident; and delineating the proportions of the human fabric, the variety obfervable in the formation of fome of them, and the tafte of different nations in their ideas of perfonal beauty. In this part the author has confulted the moft eminent anatomical writers and lecturers whom he has read and attended, particularly the late juftly admired Dr. *Hunter.*

The

The Second has for its object the art of preventing and correcting the natural deformities of the *head*; beginning with thofe of the fkull, and parts moft obvious to fight: the hair, and its defects, in refpect of colour, quantity, ftrength, &c. Then the face in general, in regard of air and mien; the forehead, eye-brows, eyes, nofe, cheeks, ears, mouth; the fkin, and complexion, as fubject to pimples, freckles, marks, and other accidental blemifhes.

We then treat of thofe parts that are lefs apparent, as the gums, teeth, and tongue, which clofes our review of the head.

In this part we have been fomewhat diffufe; induced thereto as well by profeffional knowledge, as by the nature of the fubject; prefcribing a very eafy and innocent method of preferving the teeth, and offering no recipes for their complaints but fuch as we are experimentally convinced are equally fimple and efficacious.

A 3   Some

[6]

Some obfervations on the tongue, lofs of voice, dumbnefs, and other relative articles, conclude the fecond book.

The THIRD has for its fubject the correction and prevention of bodily deformities :— We firft confider particularly the deformities of the fhape, with refpect to the trunk of the body, and the modes of relief. And fecondly, take a view of the extremities, the arms, hands, legs, and feet, with their various blemifhes, pointing out the moft approved and certain remedies, and extending the view to the minuter accidents of corns, warts, chilblains,—the nails, &c.

We firft confider the parts in their natural perfection, and teach the method of keeping them in that perfect ftate ; afterwards point out the deformities to which they are fubject, and lay down the means of correcting them, from thofe which affect the body and face, to thofe which the nails and hair are liable to :

In

In all which the precepts of HEBE will be found fingularly efficacious.

It may be neceffary to obferve, however, that we mean only fuch defects as cannot be concealed, and which it is in the power of the parties themfelves, or the parents of children, to prevent and correct. When, for example, we treat of the diforders of the *eye*, we do not pretend to fay in what manner a *gutta ferena* may be cured ; or how a *cataract* is to be couched : thefe require the knowledge of medicine, and the dexterity of chirurgery to manage them : and this remark muft be extended to all fimilar cafes.

The FOURTH BOOK confiders the fubject of Beauty in a new light. It points to the prefervation of that defirable quality by an attention to natural methods ; (namely, by exercife, diet, perfonal cleanlinefs, regulation of the paffions, amufements, &c.) founded on the invariable connection between perfect health and perfonal lovelinefs ; an

idea

idea which we have firſt endeavoured to eſtabliſh upon juſt grounds, before we draw any conſequences from it. And as we have had a particular view to the ſervice of the ladies in every part of this work, it is concluded by ſome medical precepts, for their ſole uſe and attention : they ariſe, indeed, from the foregoing conſiderations, and will, it is preſumed, be found of ſingular utility to thoſe who reſide at a diſtance from the capital, or are otherwiſe out of the reach of phyſical advice ; beſides offering the means of reſtoration to health, without injuring their delicacy by a communication of their feelings to any perſon living, or even mentioning the nature or cauſe of their diſeaſe.

The ingredients of the many uſeful recipes, which are diſperſed throughout the work, are all innocent and ſimple, can be purchaſed at much leſs expence than what is paid for a ſingle ready-made compoſition ; the effects whereof at beſt are uncertain, and often deſtructive ;

ſtructive ; while ours are uniformly rendered ſubſervient to the preſervation and improvement of *health* as well as *beauty.*

We have, indeed, been particularly ſolicitous to give ſuch preparations as are at leaſt totally devoid of every pernicious quality, and of directing the moſt effectual means for improving and preſerving the complexion, without having recourſe to any baneful methods of diſguiſing it : for with reſpect to *paints* and *rouges,* we can juſtly ſay, after having carefully analyſed all the coſmetics which have been impoſed upon the world under that denomination, that there is not one to be found, which is not abſolutely incapable, either from the texture, or the quality of its ingredients, to anſwer ſafely or effectually, the purpoſe for which it was intended.

If the ſubſtance is a powder, and dry, it may exhibit a higher complexion, but can never reflect that poliſhed clearneſs attendant on a delicate ſkin. If, on the other hand, it

is

is plaftic and adhefive, it affords a more
fhining varnifh, but totally ftops the perfpiration ; and if fpread over a confiderable furface, may, in time, produce fuch diforders
as it is impoffible to extirpate. The indif-
penfible exhalations of the vital fluid are de-
tained ; and let the ladies beware, left in the
triumph of fuperlative beauty, they fall a fa-
crifice to the ambition of futile allurements.
Let not falfe refinement induce them to deftroy that ineftimable blefling, *Health*, which
alone can give fragrance to the lip, bloom
to the countenance, and luftre to the eye.

But could this treacherous art even be
practifed with impunity, what pleafure can
it poffibly yield ?—Can it ever infpire the
foul with that confcious delight which refults
from the poffeffion of native charms ?—Can
it ever elude the keen, the penetrating gaze
of lovers ?—It may ;—but fhort will be the
triumph of impofture ;—and when detected,
—adieu to love and happinefs. Never,
therefore,

therefore, attempt to increase the bloom of youth, by methods so inadequate and destructive to all gratification.

If any thing we can say on this subject shall have a happy tendency to rescue beauty from the hands of empiricism, and mark the nice distinction by which its charms may be either improved or fatally diminished; our labour will be well rewarded.

There will be little need to urge the cultivation of personal charms upon the principle of a duty. Beauty is so amiable a personal endowment, and so principal an object in attracting the affection of both sexes, that the improvement and preservation of it will always command the attention of the elegant and refined part of mankind.

In proportion as the effects of beauty are felt and experienced, the cultivation of it has been attended to. And in most parts of Greece, in Turkey, and in Circassia, where the exquisite beauty of the women even surpasses

passes

paffes the moft luxuriant imagination, the prefervation of their charms has always been the chief object of their regard ; and certainly in no parts of the world is the cofmetic art either fo well known, or fo carefully prac- ·tifed, as in thofe countries ; where it is much more the care of the parents to model the faces of their children to the ftandard of perfection, than to polifh their minds, or culti-· vate their morals.

In thofe fertile and happy regions of the earth, the delighted mothers * may be feen daily bending the eye-brows of their little offspring into a beautiful arch, while, during the tafk of maternal fondnefs, the fmiling prattlers exult at the profpect of their future charms, and kifs with filial ardour the hands that form them for tranfport.

Though the arts of embellifhing the perfon, and the defire of engaging the admiration of the men, have in fact been pretty

similar

* Vide Dr. Chandler's Travels through Greece, &c.

fimilar among the ladies in all ages and countries ; yet we have a peculiar *penchant* for tracing fuch cuftoms among a people to whom we have been fo much indebted for our arts, fciences, and our beft notions of polifhed life. Under this idea, therefore, it may not be a difagreeable profpect to take a view, *en paffant*, of the toilette of the Grecian dames.

Some writers have been very diligent in collecting the articles which adminifter to the adjuftment of a lady's drefs—and behold the lift !

" The razor, fciffars, wax, nitre, falfe hair, fringes, lace, mitres, (a fort of fcarf or fafh) ribbands, and the pumice ftone, (formerly ufed to polifh the fkin, now for the feet only) white lead, pomatum, the crown, paints of various colours, the necklace, the fmart undrefs, hellebore, fillets, bands, the girdle, buckle, tunic, the hoop-petticoat, ear-rings, trinkets, the fly-cap, little rofes, clafps, gold

B   chains,

chains, the feal, fcarf, tippet, veil, rings, fmelling-bottles, with a thoufand other particulars, which it is impoffible for the moft exact memory to retain."

However long the catalogue, the modern dames of Greece have not fuffered one *item* to be ftruck out of it.

It muft be confeffed, that the very minute refearches into coquetry is chiefly to be attributed to thofe whofe occupation makes it neceffary for them to drefs with all poffible excitements to captivate the men ; and that 'women of this clafs have peculiar allurements of drefs to excite loofe ideas. But it muft be owned alfo, that women of character in modern Greece, as well as in modern Britain, follow their example in that particular but too often. In one refpect, however, the married ladies differ materially from many of our fair countrywomen,—that the former very commonly exert their utmoft fkill in drefs, without the leaft intention of going abroad,

or

or even being feen by any ftranger, but folely to indulge their own, and their hufband's fancy; in whofe abfence the generality of Grecian wives conftantly neglect every kind of ornament in drefs.

The extravagance of female ornaments often excited the refentment of the holy fathers of the church; and to have a complete idea of the excefs to which the women of Greece formerly carried their luxury, it will be neceffary to read the declamations of St: John Chryfoftom againft the women of his times: —declamations, however, which were imitated, and poured forth with equal refentment againft the ladies of Britain by our own clergy not a century and a half ago.

" Befides their ear-rings, fays he, they " have other ornaments for the extremity of " the cheek : their faces befmeared with " paint, and even their eye-lids not exempt " from it. They wear petticoats netted with " gold, and their necklaces are likewife all

" gold:

" gold :—upon their hands they wear plates
" of the fame metal. Their fhoes are of
" filk or velvet, glittering with embroidery,
" and terminate in a point. They ride in
" chariots, drawn by white mules, and are
" followed by a troop of maidens and fer-
" vants."

We conclude thefe remarks on the drefs
and arts of the Grecian dames, with obferving their enthufiaftic paffion for *black-eyes,**
in this partiality they are followed by the
Parifian ladies, who, perhaps, have borrowed
from the Greeks the cuftom of painting the
eye-brows and the hairs of the eye-lids of a
black colour ; for which they ufe a preparation of antimony and gall-nut.

Nor were ever female arts carried to a
greater height among the Grecian dames than
among the Parifian ladies, who certainly have
a much better apology, as being the leaft
favoured

* Homer characterizes a fine girl to be, " a beauty
" with languifhing black eyes."

favoured by nature of any women on the European continent. But as Pope juftly obferves, that a deficiency of underftanding is ufually fupplied by an ample portion of pride, fo the little fhare of perfonal charms poffeffed by the French ladies, is recompenfed to them by an unparalleled degree of *vanity* ; and they are fully perfuaded, that the genius of tafte and elegance in *drefs*, and every ornament wherewith invention continues to grace the human frame, belongs to them with an exclufive right : and *that* vanity would be highly offended, were a foreigner to difpute their fupremacy on this point. And though they make a virtue of neceffity, by yielding the palm of beauty and comelinefs to the Britifh fair ; yet they ftill tenacioufly challenge the fuperiority in all other endowments : to fupport which, they alledge the univerfal confent of other nations, in adopting their example in the above refpects ; yet the imitation of any mode is no more a proof of

the.

the imitator's approbation, than of the pro-
priety of the mode itfelf.

The difcuffion of this point would carry us
much beyond the bounds of a preface ; which
we cannot however clofe, without acknow-
ledging our obligations to many medical writers, who have occafionally condefcended to
drop hints on the fubject—but to no one
particularly fo much as Monf.Andry, late profeffor of medicine in the Royal College, and
fenior Dean of the Faculty at Paris.

LONDON,
MARCH, 1784.

TABLE

TABLE

O F

CONTENTS.

BOOK I.

Neck

B O O K II.

Of

CONTENTS.

BOOK

BOOK III.

BOOK IV.

HEBE;

H E B E.

B O O K I.

A general Description of the external Parts of the Human Body.

ANATOMISTS have ufually divided the body into the trunk, and extremities: the trunk is fupported by the fpine or back-bone, and comprehends three cavities: *viz.* the *head*, called the upper cavity, which is fupported by the neck; the *thorax*, or cheft, called the middle cavity; and the *belly*, properly fo called, but generally denominated the lower cavity.

The extremities are the *arms* and *legs*. Each of thefe is divided into a great many other parts, which we fhall name and defcribe in order, in refpect of their external appearance.

The head or upper cavity, which is the firft part of the trunk, comprehends, externally, the *cranium* or fkull; the *hairy fcalp*, or covering of the fkull; and the *face*.

The *cranium* is that bony cafe in which the brain is inclofed.

B The

The *hairy scalp* includes all that part of the head upon which the hair grows: that is to fay, the upper and hind parts of it, and the fides. The upper part of the head begins at the top of the forehead, and is called the *fynciput*; the hinder part begins at the crown of the head, and is called the *occiput*. On the fides of the head, between the eyes and the ears, are the two temples, which make a part of the *occiput*. The temporal bone is the weakeft of all the others in the head ; and hence it is, that wounds in that part are fo frequently mortal. Here, too, the firft indications of old age appear, by the hair on this part becoming grey or white.

The *face* is compofed of thofe parts which make the fore part of the head, as the brow, the eye-brows, the eye-lids, the eyes, the nofe, the ears, the cheeks, the lips, and the chin ; to which may be added the fkin, the covering of the whole; the colour, texture, and delicacy whereof is an effential ingredient in the compofition of beauty.

That fpace from the eye-brows, upward, to the beginning of the *fynciput*, is called the *front* ; which name, anatomifts tell us, it has obtained from a Greek word which fignifies to reafon, or to have reafon : it being chiefly by the brows that one knows when the mind is deeply employed in thinking.

At the loweft extremity of the forehead there arifes on each fide a fmall heap of hairs, ranged in form of an arch, called the eye-brows or *fupercilia*, becaufe they are placed immediately above that part of the eye which is called the *cilium*.

That part of the eye-brow which is neareft the nofe, is called the *head* of the eye-brow, the other is the *tail*. The space between the two eye-brows is named the *intercilium*.

The *eyes* considered externally, are composed of a great many parts;—the two little curtains which are placed above and below them, are called the eye-lids; the upper one is moveable, the other almost, though not absolutely fixed. They have each a small border planted with hair; which is called the *tarsus*, and the hair the *cilia*.

Each *tarsus* has a little opening at the side of the nose, through which the tears pass; these openings are called the *puncta lachrymalia*, and are the seat of that disorder in the eye called the *fistula lachrymalis*. The eye-lids join with each other towards the nose, and on the opposite side; by which union there is an angle formed on each side. The angle towards the nose is called the great angle of the eye, and the other is the lesser angle.

Within the eye-lids is inclosed a round polished body, called the eye, or the ball of the eye; a kind of telescope of infinite perfection, which transmits images in an exact and complete manner even to the bottom of it. This bottom is invested by textures of nerves, on which the image is imprinted, and by that means the sensation is produced, of which one of these textures is the immediate organ. What appears of this ball or globe, is white, with a point in the middle: the white part is called the white of the eye; and is composed of a coat, named the *tunica conjunctiva*, because it connects all the parts of the eye together. In the point in the middle of the eye, is a circle called the *iris*, from its variety of colours: and is furnished with muscular fibres, in the form of rays and cir-

cles,

cles, by means of which the *pupil* dilates and contracts itself. It dilates in the shade, and contracts when affected by a strong light. In the centre of this circle is that opening in the coats of the eye which we have just called the *pupil*.

The nose is that fleshy eminence or projection in the middle of the face, and is the external organ of smelling. The nose is divided into several parts.—The upper part between the eyes, or rather a little higher, is called the root of the nose; immediately below which is the spine or ridge; this part of the nose is all bony. To the spine is joined a gristly substance, which reaches to the end, and is called the globe of the nose; at the sides of which are two other cartilages or gristles, called the *perinæ*, or nostrils—The nostrils are separated by a small fleshy partition, called the *columna*; and underneath is the *philtrum*, a sort of furrow that divides the upper lip.

The sense of hearing is situate in the ear. The greatest external part of this organ consists of a large cartilage, which is the basis of the others. There are two portions, the one large and solid, called *pinna*, which is the upper part, the other small and soft, called the *lobe*, which makes the lower part. A full description of this member would lead us beyond our purposed limits; suffice it therefore to say, that the outward circle which touches the hair, is called the *helix*; and the other circle towards the face is called the *antihelix*: between these two circles is a cavity named the *boat*.

In the helix there is a semicircle called the *sickle*; and next to this a concavity named the *concha* or *shell*: under the *concha* is another cavity situated in the middle of the ear, which goes to the *tympanum*, and is called the *hole* or *hive*. The *lobe* is is divided into the upper and lower part ; to the latter of which pendants and ear-rings are faftened : near the cheek is a flat femi-circular eminence, called the *hircus*, which when preffed againft the ear ferves as a cover to fhut it exactly up.

Between the two cheeks is the cavity of the MOUTH, compofed externally of the lips, which are the entrance into it ; and confifting internally of the jaws, gums, teeth, and tongue. The lips are partly compofed of a foft fpungy fubftance, which fwells and fubfides on certain occafions, independant of the mufcular action, and is mixed with fat. The fubftance that forms the red borders of them, and which is extremely fenfible, is a collection of fine long villous papillæ, clofely connected together, and covered by a fine membrane.

The CHIN is the anterior part of the lower face : it has underneath it a flefhy part coming from the neck, called the *buccula*, or little gorge.

Along the gums of the upper and lower jaw there is a row of fmall white hard bones, which not only ferve as an ornament to the mouth, but are alfo of great ufe in chewing our food, and affifting our pronunciation :—thefe are the *teeth*. In adu'ts, or grown-up perfons, they are generally thirty fix in number, *viz.* fixteen in each jaw. Of thefe there are two fore-teeth in the front of the upper, and the fame number in the front of the lower jaw ; thefe are called *incifores*, or cutters, from their employment, which is to cut or break the fo.id food.

Next to the *incifores* are two very fharp teeth, one adjoining each of the above, called the *caninæ*, becaufe they are pointed like dogs teeth.—The two next, one adjoining each of the former, are the *eye-teeth*. The eye-teeth are fucceeded by the

four

four *small double teeth*, or *small molares* or *grinders* ;
two on each fide behind each of the eye-teeth ;
with two roots, though frequently fo connected
as to feem but one. Adjoining to thefe, are the
four *large double teeth*, two on each fide, having
three roots. Laftly, the *dentes fapientiæ*, or teeth
of wifdom, which feldom pufh out till about one-
and-twenty ; they have three roots, which are
fhorter than any other, · and generally connected through their whole fubftance. The
teeth in each jaw correfpond in fhape and number,
and are diftinguifhed by the fame titles ; except
that the large double teeth, and the *dentes fapientiæ* in the under jaw, have only two roots ; and
the four front teeth in the under jaw being all of
a fize or nearly fo, and fmaller than the four front
teeth in the upper jaw.

The next divifion of the fubject leads us to de-
lineate the external parts of the cheft.

The *neck* is commonly looked upon as a part
of the cheft, being that pillar which fupports the
head, and the principal parts which it contains depend upon the cheft. The loweft part of the neck
in front is called the throat or gullet. In the upper part of the front of the neck is a protuberance
called *Adam's apple* ; this prominence is a part of
the larynx or wind-pipe, (the inftrument of the
voice) and by its advancing forward, forms this
lump, which appears much more plainly in men
than in women; the latter having large glands in
this place, that make their necks rounder, and the
gullet more full. In the action of fwallowing, this
protuberance rifes up, and afterwards defcends ;
occafioned by the defcent of the aliment forcing the
la-

larynx to afcend while the food obtains a paffage into the ftomach.

At the fore part of the bottom of the neck, are two femicircles joined together, one on the right fide, the other on the left; thefe are the *clavicles*; two little bones that form the upper part of the vault of the cheft, which begins here, and terminates behind the falfe ribs.

The *fternum* or breaft-bone, is a flat bone placed in the middle of the breaft, filling up the fpace between the extremities of the ribs on each fide; and is that part which in animals is called the *brif-ket*. The fore-part of the cheft or thorax is properly denominated the breaft; the hinder part is called the back; the bone which divides it in the middle is compofed of twelve vertebræ or joints, and the two fcapulæ or fhoulder blades: the ufe of the parts of the thorax in general is to affift refpiration and the circulation of the blood, in both fexes; and in women to the producing of milk.

In the middle and fore part of each fide of the cheft, there rife two round tumours or eminences, called the *breafts*, which are a good deal larger in women than in men. The breafts of the former are compofed of glandular bodies, interfperfed with an infinite number of veffels, which ferve for the fecretion of milk; while thofe of the latter are nothing more than fkin, flefh and fat. In general, the breafts of men ought to be fmall, and a little plain: in women, round, high and have the appearance of two globes, feparated from each other by the middle interftice. On their center ftands a little protuberance, called *papillæ* or nipple; it is encompaffed by a reddifh circle, called the *ray*, or *areola*, which is pale in young women, brown-
ifh

ifh in women with child and nurfes, and black in old age. In females, the handfomeft breafts are round, and of the form of a hemifphere ; but the beft for giving fuck are thofe that hang down a little.

The fize of the female breaft varies in different countries, and different periods of life. In youth there is fcarce any further appearance than the nipples; but they increafe infenfibly, and are ufually formed about the age of fifteen or fixteen : they continue growing till about twenty, and remain firm till after thirty ; but at about forty-five or fifty, become quite withered, and in old age there remains nothing but the teguments.

In regard of the third cavity into which the body is divided, we fhall have little more to fay here, than that from the inferior extremity of the fternum down to the thighs, is the *lower belly*, the fore part of which is named the *abdomen.*—Any further enumeration of thefe parts, would be unneceffary, and inconfiftent with the plan of this work.

Having finifhed the trunk of the body, we come now to confider the extremities, which are the *hands* and *arms*, the *thighs* and *legs*. And indeed thefe parts themfelves, as well as their names and ufes, are fo well known and underftood as to render defcription unneceffary ; and their refpective beauties and proportions will be fufficiently pointed out when we come to treat of the means of preventing or rectifying their deformities.

The *nails* are a horny fubftance growing over the ends of the fingers and toes, ferving to defend them againft injury. Three parts are to be diftinguifhed in them ; *viz.* the root, body,

and extremity :—the root is white, and like a
crefcent, the greateft part of it being hid under the
femi-lunar fold; the body of the nail is naturally
arched, tranfparent, and of the colour of the fkin
underneath. The extremity of the nail does not
adhere to any thing, and grows as often as it
is cut, in a fimilar manner with the hair; not
from the extremity, but pufhing forward from
the root.

All the external parts of the body are wrapped
up in one common covering, the *fkin*, which is
compofed of two parts : the firft is very thin, and
is called the *epidermis*, *cuticula*, or *fcarf fkin*; the
other is thicker, lies under the cuticula, and is the
cutis, or fkin properly fo called.

The *cuticula* is a compact membrane fomewhat tranfparent, and void of feeling; it covers
all the true fkin, and adheres very clofely to it :
This is the fkin which forms the bladders or blifters
occafioned by burning. It is the colour of the
cuticula which denominates the complexion.

In the fanguine difpofition the cuticula is of a
vermillion colour, or a mixture of red and white;
in the bilous temperament, this fkin is dry, and
of a yellow caft; the flegmatic, again, have it foft
and white, while the melancholic is rough, brown,
and of a leaden colour :—not that we are to imagine thefe colours belong really to the epidermis;
but only as this membrane is very thin and tranfparent, it allows the colour of the true fkin to
appear through it, in the fame manner as objects
appear through a glafs.—The ufe of this fkin is
to cover the true one, and render it fmooth; to
hinder too great a diffipation of the humours, by
the extremities of the veffels which terminate
there; but chiefly to blunt the fenfe of touch,
which

which would otherwife be too acute, and attended
with pain, if the impreffion of objects was immediately made upon the fibres and nerves which terminate therein. We fhould truly then, in Pope's
language,

"Smart and agonize at every pore."

When the epidermis becomes thick and callous,
the fenfe of touch is not fo lively, and the perfpiration is lefs free. This fkin is very thick upon
the loins, back, and extremities; but thinner
upon the face, and ftill more fo on the lips: It
is generally more difficult to be pierced by
pointed inftruments in the belly, than in the
back.

The cutis or true fkin is a kind of net, compofed
of fibres, veins, arteries and nerves. Its ufes are
various;—it furrounds, covers, and defends the
parts that lie underneath; it is the organ of feeling; and is an univerfal emunctory to the body,
cleanfing the blood of redundancies by the means
of fweat and perfpiration; while thefe in return
help to prevent the acidity or drinefs of the cutis
itfelf. Its pores are a great deal more open and
lax in fummer than in winter; and this is the reafon that the furs of animals which have been flea'd
in winter are much better than others, becaufe the hairs are more firmly rooted in the fkin
at that time.

The foregoing obfervations will be fufficient to
give an idea of the external parts of the human
body; we fhall therefore conclude the fubject
with a few general remarks on perfonal beauty.

It will be readily allowed, that many objects
may pleafe the underftanding without interefting
the fenfes; and on the other hand, agreeable fenfations

tions may be excited by objects that have no claim to the approbation of our judgment. Hence, the impoffibility of fixing a general characteriftic of beauty; for the ideas and fenfations of different perfons vary according to their different turns of mind, and habitudes of body; and the effect of objects upon thefe ideas and fenfations, vary in the fame manner: and thus arife the different opinions refpecting, not only perfonal beauty, but painting, ftatuary, and literary compofition. The beft definition we can attempt of this vague idea, is to fay, That beauty is that pleafing effect which arifes from the harmony and juftnefs of the whole compofition.

In vain do painters and anatomifts lay down rules and proportions for beauty: the moft charming faces, and moft elegant forms frequently, nay generally deviate from thefe eftablifhed proportions; while many, in whom fuch proportions may be moft accurately obferved, are far from being agreeable, much lefs beautiful. Inftead therefore of telling the reader, that the head with the neck make a fixth part of the body,—that the meafure of the face is the length of the palm of the hand, &c. we fhall point out the conformation of the parts of the body, confidered feparately, in fuch objects as are generally allowed to be beautiful.

The head, then, ought to be rather large than otherwife; of an oval figure, flat on the fides, and moderately prominent both before and behind.

The face fhould be longer than it is broad, and have fomething of a *relievo* or projection. Among the ancients, long faces were efteemed the moft beautiful, as is evident from their ftatues; and the face of our Saviour is reprefented very long in all the ancient pictures.

The

The forehead ought to be somewhat high and prominent, but very gently so.

Each eye-brow should form an arch, and be sufficiently adorned with hair.

The eyelids to be bordered with hair of a graceful length.

The eyes large, and well set ; the nose pretty long, with nostrils of a middling wideness ; the cheeks, full, firm, and roundish.

The mouth ought to be small.

The lips moderately pouting, and their borders of a delicate vermil tincture.

The ears ought to be small, and neatly joined to the head.

The chin a little roundish.

The teeth, which (when exposed to view) adds much to the agreeableness of the countenance, should be close set, firm, white, and rather broad than otherwise ; which I think adds to the dignity and exprefion of a countenance ; while long narrow teeth have a very unmeaning appearance.

The neck disengaged from the shoulders.

The shoulders should be plain, and without any jutting out of the scapulæ or shoulder blade.

The chest, large, full, and rising.

The arms round and fleshy, a little flat inwards, and growing gradually thicker from the wrist to the joint of the elbow.

The hands somewhat plump and long, the fingers slender, and detatched from one another, with little dimples below each joint upon the back of the hand when it is open, and little risings within the hand.

The belly ought to be higher or more raised in women than in men : and the same may be said

of

of the hips —The thighs and legs are generally thicker in women than in men, though we cannot confider this as a perfection.

The waift is more flender in women, and the haunches ftand more out ; but in men the waift is longer than in women.

The calfs of the legs fhould protrude gently;—the feet be flender, and of a middling length.

Such are the parts of the human body in objects generally reputed handfome ; and though nature varies very much in the conformation of all thefe parts, yet ftill there appears an agreement among themfelves, and an evident juftnefs and perfection in their union. Thus, fhould the waift be thick and fhort, the fame fhape will obtain in the other parts of the body ; the arms will be fhort and thick, the hands broad, and the fingers thick. A perfon whofe waift is long and flender will have the limbs fo likewife. This is undoubtedly *proportion*, but not the proportion of the rule and compafs.—For a ftatue, or a human form, may be conftructed in the moft exact proportions, and by the nicest rules of art, and yet be perfectly difagreeable.

Deformity is to be confidered, not as a total privation of beauty, but as a want of congruity in the parts, or rather an inability in them to anfwer their natural defign ; as when one arm or leg is longer than the other; when the back is hunched, when the eyes fquint, and fuch fimilar defects : which, however, are not to be oppofed as a contraft to beauty ; for the unfortunate object may, in every other part of his body, be exactly well-made, and perfectly agreeable : whereas *ug-*

C   *linefs,*

linefs, which I look upon to be the proper contraft to beauty, may exift in the human form without deformity; nor can I think the ideas neceffarily connected. Uglinefs always excites our averfion to the object in which it refides; deformity as generally calls up our commiferation. Uglinefs feems to confift in the appearance of fomething malevolent to human nature. The picture of the devil always creates horror and difguft; not from the *deformity* of either his perfon or countenance, but from the *expreffion* of malice in the latter. It is from the countenance that an object is pronounced ugly, though without the leaft deformity, or even while an exact fymmetry is preferved; for it is the expreffion of the foul that gives the difguft. If this opinion be well founded, it is eafier to become beautiful than even to correct deformity, as we fhall prefently confider.

There can be no doubt but, were we able to trace things to their firft principles, we fhould find that there are different *orders of beauty*, as well as of *architecture*; and it may be truly affirmed, that nature having obferved thefe rules, the moft unhandfome face in the world in our eyes, is as perfect and regular as that which we think the beft proportioned and moft beautiful. The *volute*, and other ornaments of the *Ionic* order, are beautiful in themfelves, and at the top of an Ionic pillar; but would be a monftrous irregularity in the *Tufcan*: the flat nofe and little eyes of a Chinefe, may doubtlefs be handfome on a Chinefe countenance; but tranfplant them to the face of an Englifh woman, and they inftantly become a deformity.

I cannot avoid one remark more on this fubject, which is not unworthy of attention; namely, that
every

every face is formed in fuch a manner, that however difagreeable it may appear, (provided it has
not been disfigured by accident) it is impoffible to
make any alteration in it, or to make any fingle
part more beautiful, without rendering the whole
ftill more unhandfome.—For example, he who
fhould attempt to lengthen the nofe of a perfon,
naturally fhort, would only introduce a real deformity ; the feature thus lengthened would no
longer be proportioned to the other parts of the
face, which being of a certain largenefs, and having certain elevations or depreffions, require that
the nofe fhould be proportioned to them, however
it may deviate from the painter's ftandard of ideal
beauty. Hence we may learn, not to regard
many things as deformities, becaufe differing from
our tafte and habit, when they may, in reality, be
perfections, though in an order, or a clafs of beauty, we are not fufficiently acquainted with.

We fhall take no farther notice of the different
taftes which influence mankind in different regions
of the world, but without condemning any of them,
proceed, and confine ourfelves to the confidera-
tion of thofe forms which are generally looked
upon as effentia's of beauty in our own country.

HEBE.

H E B E.

B O O K II.

Of the Deformities of the Head.

THE head, as already obferved in Book I.
includes the fkull, the hair, and the face: the
fkull is the cafe of the brain ; the hair is the covering of this cafe; and the face is a compofition
of thofe parts which conftitute the whole fore-part
of the head.

Hence we have the deformities of three parts
to treat of ;—firft, thofe which affect the head, with
refpect to the *cranium* or fkull; fecondly, thofe with
refpect to the hair; and thirdly, thofe of the face.

Deformities of the Head with refpect to the Skull.

The head, to be well-fhaped, ought to be round-
ifh ; and, when meafured, fomewhat horizontally
long ; fwelling out a little both before and behind,
and pretty flat on the fides. This is the natural
figure of the fkull ; though it is frequently fpoiled
by the manner in which children are treated. The
beft method to preferve the heads of children well
fhaped, is to make ufe of nothing that may con-
ftrain that fhape ; but leave it entirely to the difpofition of nature. By ftriving to mould the head
into any certain figure, we confine the brain, and

run

run the rifk of difplacing the organs of fenfation, which may produce very fatal effects upon the mind. Let the head, then, be left entirely to its natural figure ; unlefs, by fome accident it has been deformed ; in which cafe it may be remedied by the application of foft bandages, without any other force.

The head of an infant will take almoft any fhape, according to the preffure it fuffers ; and from thence proceeds the difference which is found among people of different countries, with refpect to the figure of the head. In France and England, children are generally laid to fleep upon their fides, whereby the temples are compreffed, and the head affumes a form fomewhat long. In Germany again, the heads of their children are broad behind; as they are commonly laid to fleep upon their backs, with their hands tied to the fides of the cradle. And indeed almoft every nation has peculiar modes of forming this part.

Care fhould be taken of the manner of combing the heads of children ; as by neglecting to comb them equally and gently, they frequently affume a wrong fhape.

The varieties of fize in the head, proceeds from the ftronger or weaker efforts which the blood, contained in the veffels of the brain, makes to expand itfelf, while the child is yet in the womb, and the *cranium* very tender. And though a head uncommonly large, or diminutively fmall, is doubtlefs a deformity, yet it is an irremediable one ; unlefs attended to during the time of pregnancy. For women with child, who live high, and drink much wine, render the blood of the fœtus too active, and thereby may occafion the firft of thefe defects. While others, who drink only water, or

weak

weak liquors, and live poorly and low, by dimi-
nifhing the force of circulation in the blood, give
rife to the other deformity.

A conclufion in favour of a perfon's judgment is
frequently drawn from the fize of his head, but with
what juftice we pretend not to determine : though,
as we have obferved the fmallnefs of the head to
be occafioned by the weak impulfe of the blood,
it may not be an unfair furmife, that fuch whofe
heads are remarkably fmall, are likewife incapable
of that ftrong application, and intenfe thought,
which are the ufual characteriftics of genius.

As it is in the ftate of pregnancy alone that fuch
imperfections can be remedied, women in that
condition ought to be particularly attentive to
their diet, obferving a due medium in the quality
of their food, and guarding themfelves againft inordinate paffions, which agitate the blood and fpirits ; and no lefs fo from too great indolence
and inactivity.

Of the Hair.

The hair is a fort of tegument or covering for
the greateft part of animals ; it is found all
over the human body, except the foles of the
feet, and the palms of the hands. It properly lives,
and receives nutriment to diftend it, like the other
parts of the body ; though its growth is fomewhat
of a different kind, and not immediately derived
therefrom; but growing like plants out of the earth ;
or as fome plants fhoot from the parts of others,
from which, though they draw nutriment, each
has its diftinct life and œconomy.

Viewed through a microfcope, hairs appear to be
hollow, and furnifhed with a multitude of veffels;
and however fmooth they may feem to the naked
eye,

eye, yet the microfcope fhews them knotted like fome foits of grafs, or like a ftalk of oats, and fending out branches from their joints.

The branching of the hair is particularly vifible at the extremities, by the help of a glafs; for it is very apt to fplit, efpecially if worn too long, or kept too dry, and appear like a brufh.

The fize of the hairs depends upon the pores they iffue from ; if thefe be fine, thofe are fmall ; if the pores are ftraight, the hairs are fo too ; and if they are oblique, the hair is curled.

The length of the hair depends upon the quantity of the humour that feeds it ; (which is certainly of a more fimple kind than any of the other humours of the body, for hair will vegetate long after death, when all the other parts and humours are corrupted ;) and the colour, on the quality of that humour ; whence at different periods of life the colour ufually varies.

The merit of good hair confifts in its being well fed, and neither too coarfe, nor too flender.

A fine head of hair is generally confidered as a neceffary appendage, or indeed as an effential part of beauty, efpecially in the ladies ; and though this depends very much upon the natural temperament of the body, yet it may be certainly improved by the affiftance of art. Daily combing, frequent dreffing, and the ufe of plain, *unadulterated* ftarch powder, with fimple pomatum, will contribute more to its nourifhment and prefervation, than all the boafted preparations of perfumery. Application of hot irons is always prejudicial; and much frizzing will finally tear it all from the head.

Pomatums and powders for the hair may generally be purchafed cheaper, at leaft more conveniently,

ently, than they can be made; but as many readers might think a treatife of this kind deficient, that did not give recipes for fuch compofitions, we offer the following as fome of the beft that can be prepared.

Pomatum for the Hair.

Cut a fufficient quantity of hog's cheek into fmall pieces, fteep it fix or eight days in clean water, which muft be changed three times a-day; and every time the water is changed, let the flefh be ftirred with a fpatula, or the fhank of a filver tablefpoon ;—drain the flefh dry, and putting it into a clean earthen pipkin, with a pint of rofe water, and a lemon ftuck with cloves, fimmer them over the fire till the fkim looks reddifh, which take off ; remove the pipkin from the fire, and ftrain the liquor. When it has cooled, take off the fat, beat it feveral times well with cold water, till thoroughly purified, ufing rofe-water the laft time inftead of common ; drain the pomatum from the water, and fcent it with any perfume to your choice, as effence of bergamot, lemon, &c.

This is an elegant and excellent compofition for almoft every cofmetic purpofe; but particularly for the hair, which it nourifhes, ftrei gthens, preferves, and thickens, and in that refpect feems a natural pabulum or food.

The beft ftarch dried is the bafis of all hair powders, and in this fimple ftate is doubtlefs nourifhing to the hair ; but it is too generally adulterated with pernicious ingredients, fuch as unflaked lime, dried bones, or bones calcined to whitenefs, fhells of fifh calcined, and worm-eaten, or rotten wood, which are fifted through a fine hair fieve, after they have been beaten to powder. The following

is

is the method of preparing *The common white powder.*

Take four pounds of ftarch, half a pound of Florentine orrice root, fix cuttle-fifh bones, ox and fheep bones, calcined to whitenefs, of each a handful ;—beat them into powder, and fift it for ufe.

The Florentine orrice root is the ufual perfume, which naturally poffeffes a violet fmell. The whiteft and foundeft roots muft be made choice of ; and are to be powdered as fine as poffible, which can only be done during the fummer.

The following powder ftands highly recommended for promoting the regeneration of the hair, and ftrengthening and nourifhing its roots.

Take roots of calamus aromaticus, (or fweet flag) and red rofes dried, of each an ounce and a half ; gum Benjamin, an ounce ; aloes wood, three quarters of an ounce ; bean flour, and Florentine orrice root, of each half a pound ; mix them all together, and reduce them to a fine powder.—You may add, if agreeable, a few grains of mufk or civet.

Though every perfon does not poffefs a *fine head of hair,* yet there are very few who, by taking a little pains, may not preferve it from certain defects, that are very obfervable, fuch as, 1. the hair falling off ; 2. becoming forky and fplitting ; 3. being eat away by ruft.

The falling off of the hair is generally the confequence of the cavities in which the roots are lodged becoming too large. This is the reafon that

most

moſt old people are bald ; for in old age, the cavities thro' which the roots of the hair iſſue, (as well as thoſe which receive the roots of the teeth) acquire a larger diameter, whence being at too much liberty, the hair ſheds, or falls off. It is remarked alſo, that the hair frequently falls off after certain diſeaſes, as fevers, ſmall-pox, &c, theſe diſeaſes being accompanied with profuſe ſweats, or other ſymptoms, which enlarge the cavities of the hair. This cauſe being explained, it follows, that there can be no better method employed to prevent the hair falling off, than having recourſe to ſuch things as ſtraiten the pores whence they iſſue. It has been recommended to waſh the head at times with a little verjuice. The juice of onions produce the ſame effect: and in Denmark, 'tis ſaid, they make their horſes tails grow very long, by uſing combs ſoaked in a decoction of onions.

We may here obſerve, that as no medicine will produce the ſame effect upon every conſtitution, ſo in the coſmetic art, it may be ſometimes neceſſary to try various methods to obtain our deſire. The following preparations, however, all ſtand recommended upon the baſis of experience.

1. Powder your head with bruiſed parſley-ſeed, at night, once in two or three months, and the hair will never fall off.

2. To quicken the growth of your hair, dip your comb every morning in the expreſſed juice of nettles, and comb the hair the wrong way. This expedient will ſurpriſingly quicken its growth.

3. After ſhaving the head, foment it frequently with a decoction of wormwood, ſouthern-wood, ſage, betony, vervain, marjoram, myrtle, roſes, dill, and roſemary.

4. Take

4. Take the tops of hemp as foon as the plants appear above ground, and infufe them in water twenty-four hours. Dip the teeth of your comb in this fluid every morning when combing the head, and it will certainly quicken the growth of the hair.

5. The following liniment is well calculated to anfwer the fame intention.

Take fix drams of labdanum, two ounces of bear's greafe, half an ounce of honey, three drams of powdered fouthern-wood, a dram and a half of the afhes of calamus aromaticus, with a fufficient quantity of the oil of fweet almonds to make it into a liniment, nearly of the confiftence of pomatum.

6. We fhall conclude with the following compound oil for the fame intention; which very quickly makes the hair fhoot out.

Take half a pound of green fouthern-wood bruifed, boil it in a pint and a half of fweet oil, and half a pint of red wine; when fufficiently boiled, remove it from the fire, and ftrain the liquor through a linen bag; repeat this operation three times with frefh fouthern-wood; the laft time add to the ftrained liquor two ounces of bear's greafe.

The hairs are apt to fplit in the end into two or three fibres, which may be feparated by a dextrous hand into as many fmall hairs, from the end to the root. This forkednefs of the hairs proceeds moft commonly from negligence, and want of cutting; though it may fometimes be caufed by an acrid, corrofive humour, furnifhed by the blood; as is particularly obfervable in fcorbutic, and other acrimonious diforders.

To

To correct and prevent this deformity, it is neceffary, firft, to have the ends of the hair frequently cut; fecondly, to wafh it with a little ox-
gall diluted with water. But if proceeding from
any diftemperature in the blood, fuch internal medicines muft be had recourfe to, as are adapted to
purify and fweeten the humours : for example,
decoctions of faffafras, farfaparilla, and efpecially
China root; a tea of which is prepared by infufing two drams of the root in about a quart of cold
water, and leaving it to foak four or five hours,
when it may be ufed as a common drink, alone, or
mixed with a little wine. It has no tafte, and is
very effectual for blunting that acrimony of the
blood which is tranfmitted to the hair.

The colour of the hair proceeds, as was before
obferved, from the predominant humour which
nourifhes it : when nourifhed by the red parts of
the blood, the hair inclines to a red glowing colour; when fed by a thin bile, it is flaxen ; if the
bile is pretty rich, the hair is generally black, or
of a chefnut colour; and when a phlegmatic humour is predominant, the hair ufually is white.

As the proportion of thefe humours are various
in human bodies, the diverfity of colours occafioned thereby, from white to flaxen, red, chefnut,
and black, will vary accordingly. Phyfical writers feem in general of opinion, that in infancy
the hair is nourifhed with a thin bile, whence it is
for the moft part of a flaxen colour. In youth,
or in proportion as children advance to years of
puberty, the hair derives its nutriment from a
richer bile, and gradually becomes darker : while
in old age, its fupply of food is chiefly drawn from
phlegmatic humours, or that thin, pituitous part
of

of the blood called the lymph, and thence becomes white. Though this whitenefs may be afcribed to another caufe ; namely, that, as age advances, and the juices are nearly exhaufted, it may happen to the hair from not receiving fufficient fupport, as to corn, which becomes white when the roots no longer convey the accuftomed juices and nourifhment.

Clofe application to ftudy, and very intenfe thinking, or a melancholic and gloomy habit of mind, either natural or acquired, will produce the fame effects upon the hair as old age ; great anxiety, and exceffive grief, which, as well as the foregoing caufes, confume the ftrength and exhauft the fpirits, are attended with the fame confequences ; and hiftory is not wanting in examples of people, who have become fuddenly greyhaired, when under the impreffion of great impending danger, or under the influence of violent grief.

It is ufual, in fpeaking of people of a grave, thoughtful difpofition, (which is ordinarily the companion of dark hair and complexion) to fay that they are melancholy ; or that their *bile is black* ; anatomy, however, has not confirmed the fact. On the contrary it may be affirmed, that when the bile is of a pretty dark colour, the perfon has a better temperament than ordinary. This is the reafon that in the choice of a nurfe, we always prefer thofe who have dark-coloured hair. Befides, it is a very common opinion among phyficians, that the milk of black cows is wholefomer than that of others.

To change the colour of the hair is certainly difficult, though by no means impoffible. When the hair is white from old age, it is common to

ufe

uſe a leaden comb, to make it darker; and the ſame expedient is often practiſed with red hair. This method, however, makes no radical change of the colour, and only diſguiſes it for ſome time; the true colour always returning, unleſs perpetual recourſe is had to the lead.

When the hair is grey in young people, or indeed of any diſagreeable colour, it may be corrected, or changed, though not without much trouble and patience. The moſt certain way of accompliſhing this end, is by cutting off the hair as cloſe to the ſkin as poſſible, and then waſhing the nead with any of the following decoctions, ſo that the remedy may penetrate the deeper into the roots of the hair; and afterwards, in proportion as the hair grows, more care ought to be taken in waſhing the head, which method muſt be continued for ſeveral weeks.——If theſe do not abſolutely change the colour, they will at leaſt do much better than a leaden comb.

Decoctions of night-ſhade, mugwort, arſeſmart, germander, colombine, penny-royal, or the root of turmerick; the leaves of the wild vine change the hairs black, and prevent their falling off; burnt cork, roots of the holm-oak, and caper tree, barks of willow, walnut tree, and pomegranate; leaves of artichoaks, the mulberry-tree, fig-tree, raſberry-buſh; ſheils of beans, gall, and cypreſs-nuts; leaves of myrtle; green ſhells of walnuts, ivy-berries, cockle, and red beet ſeeds, and poppy flowers. Any of theſe ingredients may be boiled in rain-water, wine, or vinegar, with the addition of ſome cephalic plant, as ſage, marjoram, balm, betony, clove-july flowers, &c.

1. Com-

1. *Compoſition to change Hair Black.*

Firſt, waſh your head with ſpring water, then dip your comb in oil of tartar, and comb yourſelf in the ſun : repeat this operation three times a day for the courſe of eight or ten days, at the expiration of which time the hair will be of a fine black : to give it a delightful perfume, anoint with a little oil of Benjamin.

2. *Another Method.*

Take oils of coſtus and myrtle, of each an ounce and a half ; mix them well in a marble mortar, adding liquid pitch, expreſſed juice of walnut-trees, and gum labdanum, each half an ounce ; gall-nuts, black-lead, and frankincenſe, each a dram ; with a ſufficient quantity of the mucilage of gum-arabic, (made with a decoction of gall-nuts) to make it into an ointment, with which anoint the hair.

The following is perhaps as eaſy, cheap, and efficacious a method of changing the colour of hair, as any ever invented, and has been frequently advertiſed, and ſold at the *moderate* rate of ten ſhillings a pint.

3. To two ounces of black lead finely powdered, add one ounce of ebony ſhavings ; boil them in a quart of clear water till reduced to about a pint ; filter the decoction, add a little bergamot, or any other perfume, and bottle the liquid for uſe.

The beſt method of uſing ſuch liquids is by fixing a ſmall ſponge on the upper part of the comb, and dipping it in the preparation, as the hair will thus be more effectually wet and tinged, than by the comb alone.

D 2   Red,

Red, or fandy-coloured hair may in a very fhort
time be changed to a beautiful flaxen by the affiftance of the following compofition.

4. Take a quart of lye prepared from the afhes of
vine twigs; briony, celandine roots, and tur-
meric, of each half an ounce; faffron and lily
roots, of each two drams; flowers of mullein
yellow ftechas, broom, and St. John's wort,
each a dram; boil thefe ingredients together, and
ftrain off the liquor.

It muft be obferved, that as the hair does not
fhoot out from the extremities, but from the
roots, frequent application of any of the foregoing
compofitions is neceffary, or the hair will in time
appear of two colours.

Red and yellow hair is generally looked upon
as a kind of deformity, efpecially that very coarfe
fort which is almoft of a brick colour. *Golden
locks*, however, have been a favourite theme with
poets of all countries: Milton, fpeaking of Eve,
fays

> She, as a veil, down to her flender waift
> Her unadorned *golden* treffes wore.

Horace afks his coquetifh miftrefs,

> *Cui* FLAVAM *religas comam* ?
> Pyrrha, for whom bindeft thou
> In wreaths thy *golden* hair ?

And hiftorians tell us that the original inhabitants of this ifland were diftinguifhed by their
yellow hair; though at prefent it is by no means
confidered as an ornamental or becoming colour.
The compofitions already enumerated will anfwer
every expectation in changing this colour to a
dark chefnut or black; though it may be
proper to ufe occafionally a ftrong decoction of
knot-grafs; this, by its aftringent quality, checks
the

the too great violence with which the blood is thrown into the cavities of the hair.

When the hair is much neglected, it is very apt to become rusty, as well as forked ; and a kind of scab forms at the roots, which confumes it much in the fame manner as ruft confumes iron ; or like that corrofive moifture which is fometimes found gnawing and undermining the roots of plants, when the foil is not frequently ftirred. This ruft is often fo corrofive, that the hair will fall off in fpots, juft as the hair of a muff, which has been a long time expofed to dampnefs.

This may eafily be prevented by a decent and neceffary attention to the hair, in frequently combing it : and indeed thofe ladies and gentlemen who have their hair dreffed daily, fhould yet make a point to have it often combed from the roots, to prevent the powder, pomatum, &c. from obftructing the perfpiration; a circumftance that will more readily create diforders in the head and eyes, then any quantity of hair, however great.

When this deformity has already taken place, the beft procedure is to cut off the hair entirely, and then wafh the head with a ftrong decoction of celandine, wormwood, fage, balm, and tobacco, bruifed all together, and boiled in a fufficient quantity of red wine. After wafhing the head with this decoction, a little warm, dip a linen cloth into it, which muft be applied to the head, and continued on it for two or three days.

To this may be joined the ufe of fome other of the foregoing prefcriptions ; or one of the following may prove no lefs effectual.

Take roots of a maiden vine, roots of hemp, and cores of foft cabbages, of each two handfuls ;

D 3   dry

dry and burn them, and make a lye with the afhes: after rubbing the part well with honey, wafh it with this lye three days fucceffively.

To thofe who are more fond of preparations in the form of pomatums, the following may be defervedly recommended.

Take hen's fat, oil of hempfeed, and honey, of each a quarter of a pound ; melt them together in an earthen pipkin, and keep ftirring the mixture with a wooden fpatula till cold. This pomatum, to produce the defired effect, muft be rubbed on the part eight or ten days fucceffively.

Of the FACE in general, with refpect to the Air and Mien.

An agreeable or difagreeable face confifts lefs in the particular form of the features, than in the air and caft of the whole countenance: we fee many people very homely in regard of features, who yet have a noble, agreeable, and genteel look ; while others on the contrary have beautiful faces, but a mean, difagreeable, and for-bidding appearance.

The air of the face depends upon, as it always expreffes, the fentiments of the foul. Are you defirous to poffefs a noble look, an agreeable and pleafing air?—Cultivate noble and generous fenti-ments, and thefe fentiments will appear vifible in your countenance.

People of mean birth, who in their education commonly imbibe fuch fentiments only as are low and fawning, have as generally an air of meannefs, and cringing. The face takes the impreffion of the foul, (if we may ufe the ex-preffion) and moulds itfelf thereby. When we
are

are touched with compaffion at the fight of fome pitiable object, the face, unknown even to our-felves, inftantaneoufly difcovers the fecret emotion which actuates the foul. `The cafe is fimilar with habitual fentiments. When a child is bred up in principles of honour and 'virtue, his features are formed infenfibly thereupon, and at laft become indelible, provided fuch a courfe of education is continued until his features are fettled, and maxims of honour become habitual. Tranfient fentiments can make but flight impreffions on the countenance : but confirmed by habit, in the courfe of a good or bad education, by redoubled impreffions, they imprint on the face fuch deep characters as are never to be effaced. It is this that makes the good or bad, the ugly or beautiful countenance. When a young perfon is naturally of a choleric temper, and there is no pains taken to correct this paffion in him, his face receives the impreffion of thofe clouds and frowns which anger creates; the marks of which will never difappear, but give him an air of boifterous rough-nefs even in his fofteft moments. Let reflection play her own part never fo well afterwards, though fhe may correct, and even overcome that paffionate temper, yet the rough, angry air will remain ever after, and he will carry in his look throughout life, fomething that is difpleafing to all the world.

What has been here faid of anger is equally applicable to, and may be underftood of all the other paffions : it will alfo confirm the fentiment adopted in the former book, that it is eafier to be-ftow beauty, than to correct deformity. We may juftly infer, from the foregoing remarks, that parents are the mafters of their children's coun-

tenances :—

tenances :—the face depends upon the fentiments of the mind and heart ; the fentiments upon the education ; and the education upon the parent. If the child's features are not regular, the parents cannot give them a juft regularity ; but it is in their power to form the mind and heart ; and upon the formation of thofe depends a fpecies of beauty gre.tly preferable to the r. gularity of features, or the bloom of complexion. Such reflections are fufficient to excite the vigilance of parents in many other points which equally demand their attention.

Thus much of the Face in general, we now proceed to the means of correcting the deformities of its feveral parts, fo far as come under the power of art.

Of the FOREHEAD.

The Forehead, in youth, fhould be fmooth, and without wrinkles. To prevent wrinkles in the early ftage of life, children fhould, as much as poffible, be kept in good humour, and accuftomed to a habit of ferenity :—To efface them, when contracted, the following method may be had recourfe to, but muft be continued for fome months to have any fuccefs.—Tie a bandage about the forehead, and let it remain day and night : it muft be tied pretty tight, and care taken that it does not defcend too low over the eyes, for this may bring on a heavy, clownifh look.

The Forehead is fometimes covered with hair, which comes in a point almoft down to the root of the nofe ; fhaving this only ferves to render it more luxuriant and ftrong, fo that the top of the brow, when it has been feveral times fhaved, becomes of the colour of flate, and renders the deformity more ftriking.—The beft method to hin-

der

der the production of thofe hairs, which occafion the peak, is frequently to rub the part with *dulcified spirit of falt*; a fingle drop of which, put upon the part with a fmall brufh, and then rubbed gently with a linen cloth, will effectually kill the roots of the hair, and at the end of a few weeks they will wither and fall away.

The following liniment is given by Quincey, for the fame purpofe.

Take a quarter of a pound of quick-lime, an ounce and a half of orpiment, an ounce of Florentine orrice, half an ounce of fulphur, and the fame quantity of nitre; reduce them to a fine powder, and with a pint of lye made of bean-ftalk afhes boil the whole to a proper confiftence, which may be known by dipping a feather into it; for when boiled enough, the feathery part of the quill eafily feparates from the other; add half an ounce of any aromatic effence, and mix it into an ointment, with which you may rub the hair that grows on any part of the body.

Half an hour, fays Quincey, is enough for it to lie on at a time, and when taken off, the part muft be rubbed with oil of fweet almonds; when the forenefs it occafions is over, apply it afrefh, and fo continue till it has eaten to the very roots of the hair, and made it all fhed off.

Or, Take a quarter of an ounce of gum ivy diffolved in vinegar, a dram of orpiment, a dram of ants' eggs, and two drams of gum arabic diffolved in juice of henbane, in which half an ounce of quick-lime has been boiled: make the whole into a liniment with a fufficient quantity of fowl's greafe, and apply a little to the part where you would wifh to deftroy the hair, after being clean fhaved.

No

No more vinegar is neceſſary than juſt to diſſolve the gum ivy; nor of the henbane juice than to diſſolve the gum arabic.—This is a much gentler preſcription than the foregoing, and ſcarcely leſs efficacious.

Caſes are to be met with in ſome medical writers of horny excreſcences which project from the top of the forehead. Such inſtances are indeed very rare; but when they happen, become proper objects of the ſurgeon's attention.

Children are apt to receive blows upon the forehead, either by falls, or other accidents; which ought not to be neglected, becauſe ſometimes they produce inequalities in the brow by hardening there; but are eaſily prevented by applying a ſmall plate of lead, or a halfpenny to the lump; then put a piece of linen rag, doubled a few times, and dipped in brandy, over it, with a bandage over all, and in a few days it will be well again.

Of the Eye-Brows.

The Eye-brows, to be handſome, ought to be ſufficiently furniſhed with hair; but at the ſame time to be only moderately thick. Each eye-brow ſhould form an arch upon the forehead, the hollow of which makes a ſmall vault above the eye. The head of the eye-brow ſhould be thicker than the tail; the interceil, or ſpace between the eye-brows, quite free of hair; the hair ought to be ſhort, and leave no bald ſpots; and the colour ſhould be a dark cheſnut, or black.

When the eye brows are not ſufficiently planted with hair, and you wiſh to encreaſe it, you muſt begin with ſhaving, ſo as not to leave the leaſt down upon them, and afterwards foment with
a de-

a decoction of wormwood, betony, or fage, boiled in white wine. You may afterwards ufe any of the preparations already mentioned for thickening the hair.

·If the hair falls off from the eye-brows, the following will contribute to prevent or retrieve the misfortune.

Take half an ounce of lead-filings, reduced to a very fine powder; linfeed oil an ounce and a half; powder of maiden hair, one dram ; black henbane feeds, two drams ; unguentum irrinicum, an ounce ; bruife the feeds, and make an ointment ; into which dip little flips of black filk or velvet; lay them on the eye-brows, and when you renew them, wafh the place with white wine, in which myrtle berries have been feethed.

If the eye-brows are too thick, all the help that can be made, is very carefully to clip off fome of the tops of the hairs ; an operation fo nice, that the perfons muft not venture to do it themfelves ; fhaving muft not he attempted, as it will only make them grow thicker. An application of the oil of nuts is very ferviceable in this cafe; or the eye-brows may be frequently rubbed with a lye made of the afhes of burnt cabbage.

The eye-brows are certainly moft beautiful when they form an arch ; and when they are a little ftrait, it may be thought an imperfection, though by no means a deformity. It is indeed poffible to make them arched, when very bufhy, by ufing the razor; but as the fhaving muft be frequently renewed, that practice will be foon difcovered. An application of dulcified fpirit of falt, if ufed with very great care and delicacy, may affift in this intention. [See the method under the article Forehead.

When

When the head of the eye-brow, or that part next the nofe, is too thin of hair, the defect may be eafily remedied by fhaving very fmooth, and ufing the fame means as directed for thickening the eye-brows in general.

So fluctuating is tafte, that what the ladies in the time of Ovid and Petronius employed their art to procure, is now regarded as an actual deformity ; namely, the *eye-brows joined together* ; nay, even confidered by phyfiognomifts as characteriftic of a bad difpofition :—though on a very groundlefs foundation.—In this cafe, however, the beft method of removing the deformity, is that prefcribed above for the eye-brows when too thick ; namely, a lie made of the afhes of cabbage, avoiding the ufe of the razor, for the reafon given there.

When the hair of the eye-brows lies inverted, or from the temples towards the nofe, inftead of pointing towards the former, we cannot too quickly attempt to reclaim the error. The eye-brows muft be conftantly ftroaked with the fingers from the nofe towards the temple, and continued every day for fome time ; or a tooth-brufh may be applied in the fame manner. The method is equally fimple and effectual, but ought to be made ufe of very early in life, and continued for fome time.

The hair of the eye-brows fhould be fhort and uninterrupted ; the hair be properly trimmed by a fkilful and delicate hand ; and where it is interrupted, the razor may be applied from time to time, by which, after ufing it ten or twelve times, the vacancies will be fufficiently covered with hair.

When

When the hairs of the eye-brows ſtand an end, or ſtart from each other, let them be ſhaved off a few times, taking care after ſhaving to paſs the finger frequently over them in the proper direction ;—this will ſoon make the hairs lie ſmooth without over-topping each other.

The moſt agreeable colour of the eye-brows is thought to be a black, or a dark cheſnut : the moſt diſagreeable, red.—To procure the former, and diſguiſe the latter colour, you muſt ſet fire to about a dram of frankincenſe and maſtick, receiving the ſmoke upon the inſide of a ſilver ſpoon, paſſed backwards and forwards over the flame ; with the ſoot thus collected, rub the eye-brows, taking care not to touch the adjoining parts, leſt you ſhould black them ; for this is a very tenacious colour, and will not eaſily come off.

Or, you may waſh the eye-brows with a decoction of gall-nuts, then wet them with a hair pencil dipped in a ſolution of green vitriol, in which a little gum-arabic has been diſſolved :—when dry, they will appear of a beautiful black colour.

The former preſcription has this advantage, that the colour will not come off by ſweating.—It may be neceſſary to inform the ladies, that this proceſs muſt be often repeated, as it is impoſſible to effect a radical change of colour here, as in the hair of the head, on account of waſhing, &c. the face.

We have obſerved that the arch of the eye-brows ſhould be entire, reaching from above the ſide of the noſe very near to the temple.

When this ſhape of the eye-brow is imperfect, and there is not a ſufficient diſtance between the head and tail, recourſe muſt be had to the razor,

E   and

and frequent fhaving of the part where hair is
wanting; and even when there is no hair to take
off, the operation muft be continued ; for the
action of the razor brings the nourifhing juice to
the parts, revives the roots of the hair, and en-
larges their cavities when too clofely locked up.
We fpeak this under the fuppofition that fuch
roots really exift ; otherwife no power of art can
produce them.

The arch of the eye-brow may be too much ele-
vated, which gives an air of boldnefs and affu-
rance, particularly d.fagreeable in the ladies : and
this defect is beyond the power of art to reform.
Yet it may be in fome degree palliated by affuming
a modeft, downcaft look, which attention will
foon render habitual.

There is fometimes a deficiency of *one* or *both* of
the eye-brows : the latter is fo fmall a deformity,
and fo little obferved, that it is not worth the
pains to correct it. When the want of one eye-
brow only, proceeds not from a burn, or fome
other accident, or from a natural deficiency in the
fhoots of hair, it is poffible to remedy the defect.
If you have reafon to believe that the deficiency
is to be afcribed either to a fcarcity of the nourifhing humour, or to the ftraitnefs of the pores
through which the hair ought to pafs; you muft
proceed as in fimilar cafes of a deficiency of hair,
by fhaving, and afterwards wetting it with fuch
liquors as are analogous to that humour which
nature furnifhes for the nourifhment of the hair:
the natural humour appears to be an oily, water-
ifh mixture, fomewhat falt and bitter : fomething
fimilar to this may be produced by the following
compofition.

Of

Of the oils of honey, wormwood, and bitter almonds, each three drops; of the person's own
urine five drops, mix these together, make them
milk-warm, and rub the part with this liquor
several times a-day for three months, or more, till
the points of the hair begin to appear upon the
eye-brow ; and after that continue the same
method till the eye-brow is quite grown. If the
deficiency proceeds from the last-mentioned causes,
this method is the best that can be adopted, and
generally succeeds : but if the eye-brow has been
accidently destroyed, or there is a natural want
of hair-roots, we only lose labour in attempting
to correct it.

As we think it neceffary to notice every
defect, however uncommon, we cannot conclude this article without directing the means
of eradicating another deformity, namely, when
the eye-brows are double, one above another;
which however difficult, may yet be accomplished.

You must first examine which of the eye-brows
deferves best to be kept ; and when this is deter-
mined, proceed in the following manner.

Shave the eye-brow that you resolve to destroy,
and immediately after rub upon it a little dulcified
spirit of salt, by means of a very small hair-pencil,
taking especial care that none of the spirit get into
the eye, This application must be continued two
days succeffively, morning and evening, and the
third day the part must be rubbed with spirit of
wine. On the fourth, repeat the application of
the spirit of salt, but only for one day ; renew it
eight days afterwards, and then discontinue it for
at least fifteen days. If before the end of that
time you obferve the eye-brows begin to grow

again,

again, the operation muſt be entirely renewed; but a perſeverance in this method will infallibly take away the ſuperfluous eye-brow.

Of the NOSE.

There are ſeveral deformities of the Noſe which may juſtly be attributed to the negligence, or to the miſmanagement of nurſes and parents, during early infancy, and which no future care, or aſſiſtance from art, can rectify. Among theſe we may claſs, the noſe being flat or broad; turned up, reſembling a por-hook; and ſtanding awry.

The firſt is occaſioned by the nurſe preſſing too hard upon the child's noſe in blowing it, for it ought to be wiped very gently;—frequently compreſſing the noſe between the fore-finger and thumb, will help to correct this; and there is no other means which can be taken with ſafety.—By rubbing the noſe up towards the forehead, it is apt to form into a ſhape reſembling a pot-hook; its original figure is only to be recovered by paſſing the fingers every now and then upon the ridge of the noſe, from top to bottom, and preſſing the end pretty ſtrongly down; frequently, however, ſqueezing the noſtrils gently, to prevent them growing wider by the preſſure on the noſe.— When this organ is negligently thruſt awry, there is no need for any other remedy, than the aſſiſtance of the fingers in puſhing the noſe from that ſide to which it is moſt inclined.

All theſe defects muſt be corrected when the child is very young, and to accompliſh it, will be a taſk for the patience of any old woman: though maternal fondneſs will think no trouble or pains too much, which prevents a deformity in, or inſures the comelineſs and welfare of the offspring.

By

By a large nofe, I would wifh to have underftood, cne that is fo to a deformity; and which,
when hereditary, or not corrected at a very early
period in life, admits of no palliation any more
then when occafioned by a fright at the view of
monftrous mafks or pictures during the time of
pregnancy.

When, therefore, a child is born with an uncommonly large nofe, which cannot be imputed
to any of the preceding caufes, and there appears
no figns of its diminution in the courfe of fix or
feven months, it will be proper to have it
moiftened with the juice of purflane and lettice,
frefh preffed, and a little warm : the juice of beets
may likewife be fnuffed up the nofe feveral times
a day for a month together. If thefe methods
have no fuccefs in the courfe of eight or ten
weeks, the cure muft be left to nature; and there
are not wanting examples of children, who have
had the nofe deformed, as to fize, till they were
two or three years old, and yet the deformity has
afterwards vanifhed.

Other methods have, indeed, been tried; but
as they cannot be fafely recommended, we think
it our duty to omit them, except the fubjoined
fomentation, which is perfectly innocent, and
often efficacious.

Take a pint of white Champaign wine, the
ftrongeft and moft fparkling you can get, the half
of a middle fized quince, cut into three or four
piaces, two drams of rock-allum, and a handful
of pomegranate bark, (if readily procured); boil
all together for a minute or two, then cover the
veffel up clofe, and let it ftand half an hour; after
which, when about luke-warm, foak a linen rag
in

E 3

in it, which apply to the nofe; and this muft be
repeated feveral times a day for fome months

In confequence of fevere colds, an acrid ferum
will diftil through the nofe, erode the border of the
noftrils, and make them gape towards their extremity: Nature frequently fills up this opening, but
fometimes it continues for life, not excoriated, but
healed in fuch a manner, that the appearance of the
old fore ftill remains very difagreeable. It is beft
to make a fpeedy cure of this, by anointing the
noftrils with fine frefh butter, and a little of the oil
of eggs, mixed together in the palm of the hand,
and repeated feveral times.—A remedy much fuperior to any pomatums.

Sometimes the nofe is feized with a convulfive
fpafm, which makes it move involuntarily; fome
have this motion when they laugh, others when
they are vexed or angry, or intent upon any thing;
and many have it all times indifferently. This
motion of the nofe, when it has been long neglected, admits of no remedy; but it may be cured,
if means are ufed at firft. Whenever therefore
it comes on, immediately apply a linen rag
dipped in cold water to the part, which muft
be repeated feveral times. ———— Involuntary
motions, in any other part of the face, will yield
to this application, if timely ufed.

The nofe oft-times appears pricked full of
fmall holes, like the fhells of almonds. 'Tis
generally believed that thefe little holes are apart-
ments for worms, and upon this notion it is ufual
to pinch fuch places between the nails, to fqueeze
out the imaginary vermin, which are nothing elfe
than a greafy fubftance hardened in the holes.
Pinching with the nails fqeezes out this ftuff effectually; but then on the other hand, it produces
three

three very bad effects: the first is that of making the nose red; secondly, making it grow large; and thirdly, occasioning tumours to rise upon it.

The moft fuccefsful method of obliterating thefe little holes, is to rub a few drops of the oil of nutmegs with the finger, or a fmall brufh, all along the nose. This application renewed feveral times for a few weeks, foftens the pent-up matter, and makes it come out by only rubbing the nofe with a bit of linen rag: after which, a few drops of the vinegar of rofes, rubbed gently upon the nofe, fhuts up thefe little apertures, that they no longer appear.

A *Polypus* in the nofe, is a flefhy excrefcence that fometimes fills one or both noftrils, in fuch a manner, that there is no free paffage for the air; nay, frequently, it cannot obtain the leaft admittance, whereby the refpiration is prevented, the voice altered, the fpeech rendered difficult, and the nofe confiderably fwelled. Thefe excrefcences are fometimes foft; at others hard and rigid; fmall in their beginning, but gradually increafe, and often hang out of the nofe down to the lips.

This deformity is ufually fuppofed to require the affiftance of a fkilful furgeon in order to extract it; but Mr. Andry, a very diftinguifhed Phyfician of Paris, treats it in a much eafier and more agreeable method.

To cure this difeafe, fays he, we muft not go roughly to work, but proceed very gently. Some people believe that there is nothing to be done, but to cut and tear it out, while this treatment will certainly exafperate the polypus, fo as make it degenerate into a cancer.

The

The difeafe is ftill curable, whether the polypus
poffeffes the whole cavity of the nofe, or only a
part of it; though the cure is doubtlefs more difficult in the one cafe than in the other. If the whole
cavity of the nofe is not filled with the polypus,
there needs no other remedy than a little broth
made of veal and crabs, introduced milk-warm
into the nofe. This may be done by foaking a bit
of fpunge in the broth, then wring out the liquor
into the palm of the hand, and fnuff it up the
nofe:—this muft be repeated feveral times a-day
for a good many weeks together.

When the excrefcence is fo large as to fill up
the whole cavity of the nofe, the beft method even
then for removing it, is to moiften it with the
broth juft now recommended: it may be introduced by means of a fmall fyringe, between the
polypus and the fide of the nofe to which it
adheres. This muft be repeated two or three times
a day for a month, or longer, in proportion to the
obftinacy of the cafe.

Monf. Le Clerc, a well-known and celebrated
phyfical writer, obferves, that, befides the general
remedies, which are blood-letting and purgations,
with an exact regulation of diet, there are alfo
particular medicaments that dry up, and infenfibly
confume the excrefcence; as a decoction of biftort,
plantain, and pomegranate rinds, in claret wine,
which is to be fnuffed up the nofe many times in a
day; to which a little alum and honey may be added. — The patient may likewife keep chewing
a fage leaf, a little pellitory of Spain, tobacco,
or any thing of the kind, which brings the faliva
into the mouth. If the tumor does not yield to
thefe remedies, it will be neceffary to have recourfe to manual operation.

What

What generally gives occafion to the polypus, of which we are now treating, is the pulling off with the nail certain mucous fubftances that are fixed to the infide of the nofe, and form crufts there. Thefe crufts fometimes ftick fo very clofe, that if you have not patience to let them take their own time, and fall off of themfelves, (which would be in a few days) they are not to be removed without taking the fkin off the part they are attached to ; and this is generally fufficient to produce the diforder.

There grow likewife at times within the nofe, pretty long hairs, which point out at the noftrils, and being rather looked upon as unfeemly, inftead of cutting them, people frequently pull them out by the roots, that they may not be difcerned. One or other of the foregoing caufes is generally the occafion of fuch excrefcences.

Pimples frequently break out on the nofe, and caufe a difagreeable appearance ; the application of fome fuch cooling liquid as the following, will generally be fuccefsful in taking them off ; obferving at the time you ufe it to take a few dofes of any cooling purgative.

Boil together a handful of the herbs patience, and pimpernle, in a quart of water, to a pint ; and wafh the nofe with it every every day.—It may be ufed to the whole face, which it will make very clear, taking away all eruptions.

Of the Eye-Lids.

There are feveral deformities to which this feature is liable, of which we fhall proceed to take a concife review.

Sometimes the upper eye-lid is fo turned up towards the forehead, that the eye can only
be

be half clofed ; and people in this fituation, fleep with their eyes open like hares ; and hence this deformity is called the *hare-eye*. It may either proceed from a bad conformation of the eye, or be contracted by a bad cuftom which children are fuffered to acquire in the cradle, of looking always upwards ; and thus fixing the eye-lid towards the brow.

. The fame deformity may likewife proceed from. an acrid humour, falling upon the mufcular membranes of the eye-lids, and eroding them by its acrimony ; as likewife from the fcar left after an ulcer, or any hurt on this part.

When the defect in queftion proceeds from an acrimonious humour, diftilling upon the part, recourfe muft be had chiefly to internal medicines, of the fweetening and abforbent kind, as decoctions of guaiacum, farfaparilla, china-root, faffafras, &c.—Externally, you may wet a comprefs in rofe-water, and apply it to the eye-lids, taking care to renew it from time to time, fo as not to let it dry on the part.

When the deformity proceeds from a habit, contracted by the child in the cradle, of looking always upwards, nothing more is requifite than to put a fillet over his forehead, fo as quite to cover the eye-lids, and thus prevent him from looking up : obferving, before you tie the fillet, to pull the eye-lids gently downwards.

Children may either bring on or increafe this deformity by playing too frequently at fhuttle-cock, or fuch diverfions as oblige them to turn their eyes upwards.

The turning down of the lower eye-lid is a greater blemifh than the turning up of the upper one ; when this is not the effect of fome wound

of

of the eye-lid, it generally proceeds from a relaxation of the part, produced by too much moisture,
which deprives it of motion and elasticity; for
although the lower eye-lid may be looked upon
as immoveable in comparison of the other, yet it
is not absolutely so : for it moves at the same
time with the upper eye-lid ; both of them have
the same motion, which is only less sensible in the
under one, but not less real. And anatomy teaches
us, that both eye-lids have the same muscles
and the same fibres for producing this motion.
In the present case, however, the muscles are not
able to move the lower eye-lid, on account of the
too great humidity which relaxes them ; it follows
then, that to restore this motion, and strengthen
the eye-lid, recourse must be had to medicines
which evacuate the superfluous serous humours,
and afterwards make use of astringents and
strengtheners. A blister may be applied between
the shoulders, or to the nape of the neck, with
good effect.

When strengthners become necessary, you may
bathe the eye-lid frequently with plantain and
fennel water, in which a piece of hot iron has
been extinguished.

Or take sugar of lead and white vitriol, each
five grains ; rose water two ounces ; mix, and
use.

A little tumour is often produced between the
membranes of the upper eye-lid, shining, moveable, round, and hard, about the size of a pea,
hanging by a very slender stalk, and in some mea-
sure resembling the figure of a hail-stone. This
tumour is not dangerous, unless it be irritated by
improper applications. It will sometimes disappear without the use of any remedy. When applications

plications become neceffary, nothing is fo proper as fomentations in the form of fteam ; and for this purpofe the following herbs, well dried, muft be boiled in common water ; *viz.* balm, fweet-bafil, origanum, marjoram, bleffed thiftle, of each a handful ; to thefe muft be added half a handful of bay-berries, and juniper-berries, bruifed, with a fmall handful of coffee well roafted and powdered. While the decoction is hot, let the fteam be directed to the eye by the means of a funnel, taking care to keep the eye clofe fhut.

Let the decoction be again heated, and repeat the operation feveral times every day, without intermiffion, till the cure is compleated : taking care, however, not to handle the tumour too roughly, left it be rendered incurable.

There is another tumour, which grows upon either eye-lid, but moft frequently upon the upper one, foft, red, and tranfparent, which hinders the eye from opening ; it is caufed by a watery humour, extravafated between the membranes of the eye-lid. Children are very fubject to it, and unlefs great attention is paid, it may quit its indolent appearance, become very painful, and degenerate into a fiftulous ulcer ; or leave an ugly troublefome fcar upon the eye-lid. The cure of this blemifh is, by applying a poultice of mugwort, fcabious, fage, fennel, and agrimony, boiled in white wine. If, after the ufe of this cataplafm, the tumour feems difpofed to fuppurate, you muft apply another, made with common mallows, marfh-mallows, figs, camomile, faffron, and the crumbs of bread boiled in milk, and continue this till the fuppuration is brought on. The fore may be afterwards healed up with the honey of rofes, and a little tutty.

At

At the border of the eye-lid, growing upon the cilia, is frequently another small inflamed tumour, long, immovable, of the figure of a grain of barley, generally called a *hordeolum*, well known in many parts by the name of a *fly:* it begins at first with a little red swelling, which grows larger by degrees, attended with itching and heat; and after some days becomes white, and suppurates.

The *hordeolum* is without danger, if not fretted with the fingers, and for the most part heals of itself. It is frequently cured by the bare application or rubbing of the tumour with a piece of smooth gold or silver dipped in spring water: and this if applied early, is an infallible cure. But if the complaint be neglected, then the mode of cure must be suited to the circumstances that attend it: if there be an inflammation, the pulp of a roasted apple applied by way of poultice, sometimes disperses it, and at other times only abates the tumour. If it hardens, it must be opened with a launcet, and the hard flesh consumed by a liquid cauftic.

The want of the *cilia*, or hairs of the eye-lids, is less a deformity than a source of pain to the person in whom they are wanting. The most common cause of the want of these hairs, is crying too much in infancy. The tears, being a very sharp humour, destroy the roots of the hairs upon the borders of the eye-lids, nay sometimes are so acrid as to excoriate the very cheeks.

When the roots of the *cilia* are absolutely destroyed, 'tis impossible ever to produce them afresh : for notwithstanding the boasts of empirics,

F　　　　'tis

'tis no more poffible to produce hair in fuch a cafe, than to raife a plant without either root or feed. But if any part of the root of the cilia remain, and the pores through which the hairs naturally fprout are not quite effaced, there is hope of reftoring the cilia again by rubbing the borders of the eye lids with a decoction of betony, fage, lavender, balm, and origanum, with a little honey added to it.

The cilia ought to be pretty long and thick, without which the eye-lids will not look fo well, however beautiful they may otherwife be.

To make them grow long and thick, frequently anoint them with the oils of juniper and amber mixed together. Or, take thirty common flies, bruife them, and make them into a plaifter with a little turpentine diffolved in the yolk of an egg, and apply it to the eye-lid ; than which, nothing can be more excellent even to reftore the cilia.

In fome perfons there are two rows of hair upon the cilia, the one above the other, refembling the eye-brows above-mentioned, but are a greater blemifh, and at the fame time hurtful, becaufe they prick the eye, and occafion a pain and running, on which account the deformity cannot be too foon rectified. The method of curing it, is to pull out all thofe hairs that hurt the eye, with a pair of fine tweezers, which may be eafily done when the child is pretty young, provided you pull ftraight, and go gently to work.

When the hairs are pulled out, take half an ounce of frefh butter, gall of a pike, one dram ; tutty, two fcruples ; and three or four grains of camphire ; with this rub the eye-lids frequently, to prevent the hairs from growing anew. If they fhould fhoot out, they muft be plucked as before: but

but this will fcarce happen above two or three times.

In people who are grown up, the plucking of the cilia might be dangerous; the beft method, therefore, is to clip away the hairs which turn inward, with a pair of very fmall fciffars, as near to the border of the eye-lid as poffible, and afterwards to rub the part with the juice of the flowers of colt's foot, and a little milk warmed; which method ought to be frequently repeated.

Of the Eyes.

Squinting is a deformity of the eye fo well known as not to require defcription. Frequently brought on in infants, by letting them conftantly fuck at one and the fame breaft; or from placing them in the cradle, fo that they always look the fame way towards the light or window; by this repeated action, the mufcles on that fide become too ftrong to be balanced by the oppofite ones, and hence the eye looks obliquely at objects. It may be alfo caufed by convulfive motions; to which the eyes of children are internally fubject. And it may, laftly, proceed from fpafms, a palfy in fome of the mufcles of the eye, or from a defect in fome part of the retina.

A frequent fault of nurfes is, that when they want to ftill a crying child, they hold up againft its eyes a doll, a coral, or fome other toy which they make to jump about, fo that the child cannot look upon an object fo near without fquinting.

Squinting is very difficult of cure, efpecially in grown-up people, and particularly when caufed by any defect in the mufcles, or retina.

The method moft highly recommended, is to make the child view his own eyes in a looking-

glafs,

glafs, about a quarter of an hour every morning and evening for feveral days ; with this precaution, that each eye fhould look at its correfponding one in the mirror.

Thofe who are advanced in years, may be af-fifted by reading very fmall writing or print; or by infpecting very minute objects, provided they turn their eyes even, and bathe them at times with Hungary water. But this practice muft not be too clofely followed, efpecially in children, left it fhould increafe the diforder. . Nor is the difad-vantage of a child being a year or two later in learning to read, to be compared with that of running a rifque to be fquint-eyed all his life.

After all, if the fquinting is not confiderable, it may be paffed over as a defect, which often does not deferve the name of a deformity ; for there are fome fquints not at all difagreeable ; and *Ovid* praifes thofe beauties of his time who fquinted a little ; for fuch, according to him, were the eyes of *Venus*.

Si pæta eft, Veneri fimilis.
OVID DE ART. AMOR.

The following very curious cafe is extracted from the Philofophical Tranfactions of 1780, and is communicated by *Erafmus Darwin*, M. D. F. R. S.

About fix years ago, Dr. Darwin was defired to vifit the child of the Rev. Dr. Standford, in Shropfhire, to determine if any method could be devifed to cure him of fquinting : the child was then about five years old, and exceedingly tracta-ble, by which the doctor was enabled to make fe-veral ufeful obfervations upon him with great ac-curacy, and frequent repetition.

The

The child viewed every object which was prefented to him, with but one eye at a time.

If the object was prefented on his right fide,
he viewed it with his left eye; and if it was
prefented on his left fide, he viewed it with his
right eye.

When an object was held directly before him,
he turned his head a little to one fide, and obferved
it but with one eye ; namely, with that moft diftant from the object, turning away the other ;
and when he became tired with obferving it with
that eye, he turned his head the contrary way,
and obferved it with the other eye alone, with
equal facility ; but never turned the axes of both
eyes on it at the fame time.

He faw letters, which were written on bits of
paper, fo as to name them with equal eafe, and
at equal diftances, with one eye as the other.

From thefe circumftances it appeared, that there
was no defect in either eye, which is the common
caufe of fquinting, but that the difeafe was fimply
a depraved habit of moving his eyes, and might
probably be occafioned by the form of a cap or
head-drefs, which might have been too prominent
on the fide of his face, like bluffs ufed on coach-
horfes ; and might thence, in early infancy, have
made it more convenient for the child to view objects placed obliquely with the oppofite eye ; till
by habit the *mufculi adductores* were become
ftronger and more ready for motion than their an-
tagonifts.

A paper *gnomon*, or artificial nofe, was made and
fixed to a cap, and placed over his real nofe, fo as
to project an inch between his eyes ; when the
child, rather than turn his head fo far to look at

F 3 . oblique

oblique objects, immediately began to view them with that eye which was next to him.

The death of Dr. Sandford, however, prevented any further progrefs in this experiment, for the fpace of fix years: when Dr. Darwin feeing him a fecond time, obferved all the circumftances of his mode of vifion to be exactly the fame as before, except that they feemed eftablifhed by longer habit, and he could not be induced by any means to bend the axes of both his eyes on the fame object, not even for a moment.

A gnomon of thin brafs was made to ftand over his nofe, with a half circle of the fame metal to go round his temples : thefe were covered with black filk, and by means of a buckle behind his head, and a crofs piece over the crown of his head, this gnomon was managed fo as to be worn without any inconvenience, and projected before his nofe about two inches and a half. By the ufe of this gnomon he foon found it lefs inconvenient to view all oblique objects with the eye next to them, inftead of the eye to him.

After this habit was weakened by a week's ufe of the gnomon, two bits of wood, about the fize of a goofe-quill, were blackened, all but a quarter of an inch at their fummits; thefe were frequently prefented for him to look at, one being held on one fide the extremity of the gnomon, and the other on the other fide of it. As he viewed thefe, they were gradually brought forward beyond the gnomon, and then one was concealed behind the other ; by thefe means, in another week, he could bend both his eyes on the fame object for half a minute together.

By the practice of this exercife before a glafs, almoft every hour in the day, he became in another

ther week able to read for a minute together with
both his eyes directed on the fame object : and I
have no doubt (adds the writer),if he has patience
enough to prefevere in thefe efforts, but he will, in
the courfe of fome months, overcome this unfightly habit.

I fhall conclude this account with adding, that
all the other fquinting people I have had occafion
to attend to, have had one eye much lefs perfect
than the other. Thefe patients, where the difeafed
eye is not too bad, are certainly curable by covering the beft eye many hours in a day ; as by a
more frequent ufe of the weak eye, it not only
acquires a habit of turning to the objects which
the patient wifhes to fee, but gains at the fame
time a more diftinct vifion ; and the better eye
feems to lofe fomewhat in both thefe refpects,
which alfo facilitates the cure.

This evinces the abfurdity of the practice of
prohibiting thofe who have weak eyes from ufing
them ; fince the eye, as well as every other part of
the body, acquires ftrength from that degree of
exercife which is not accompanied by pain or
fatigue ; and I am induced to believe, that the
moft general caufe of fquinting in children originates from the cuftom of covering the weak eye,
which has been difeafed by any accidental caufe,
before the habit of obferving objects with both
eyes was perfectly eftablifhed.

In the conclufion of a fupplement to this cafe
(containing fome remarks on the nature of vifion,
Mr. Darwin further adds, " that by ufing the artificial nofe, the child has greatly corrected the
habit of viewing objects with the eye furtheft from
them ; and has more and more acquired the voluntary power of directing both his eyes to the

fame object, particularly if the object be not more than four or five feet diftant from him ; and will, I believe, by refolute perfeverance, entirely correct this unfightly deformity.

A wandering, unfettled eye, is what we hardly know whether to treat as a deformity, or commiferate as a misfortune ; fince a perfon of this unfettled look is too generally fuppofed, though often unjuftly, to be of as unfettled a mind. Nothing contributes more to give children wandering eyes, than expofing to their view a great huddle of objects in motion ; fuch as foldiers marching ; or a mixed multitude of people dancing and jumping, as is ufual in places of rejoicing whither children are generally carried : for it is impoffible in fuch a multiplicity of objects to view any of them at leifure, or diftinctly; this fets the eye a-wandering, till they cannot look fteadily at any thing, and the defect increafes with years ; whence you may obferve fo many people, who, while they are talking to you, feem to have their eye fixed upon you, yet in the mean time do not fee you ; they are looking at fomething elfe, one knows not what.

When a perfon becomes confcious of this misfortune, it is highly probable that reflection and perfeverance, may greatly contribute to palliate or overcome the defect : but art affords no relief.

A *fquamous,* or *fcaly eye,* is a blemifh produced by certain hard, fmall, fcaly pellicles, formed between the eye-lid and the ball of the eye, which either deftroy the fight entirely, or at leaft hurt it confiderably, and in both cafes occafion divers contorfions of the eye.

A great

A great light darting in upon the eyes, fo as to dazzle them much, and raife a commotion in the innermoft parts of the eye, is frequently the caufe of this difeafe. Befides a great many other examples which might be produced, we have a remarkable inftance of this in the perfon of St. Paul, upon whofe eyes, as the fcripture fays, there were formed fmall pellicles,refembling fcales, after he was ftruck to the ground with lightning ; and he did not recover till they were fallen off. Thofe who travel over waftes of fnow, are obliged to wear fpectacles, made of a particular fort of glafs, to defend their eyes from the dazzling luftre of the profpect, and preferve them from thofe fcales; which, when they have been of long continuance, become fo incorporated with the eye, that it requires the greateft art in the world to remove them.

'Tis no uncommon thing to expofe children's eyes to all forts of light indifferently, and even to that of the brighteft fun ; though in many cafes, one fingle ray of the fun darted ftrongly upon the eyes of a child, may dazzle him to fuch a degree, as to deprive him of fight entirely.

Another very neceffary precaution is, never to fuffer children to lay oppofite to a ftrong light ; but to put a thin curtain between them and the place from whence it comes ; or to place them in fuch a manner as they may have the light on their back, or on one fide. The fame precaution ought to be obferved by teachers, to prevent the light coming full on the faces of their pupils, which circumftance is of itfelf fufficient to render their eyes fcaly, and greatly injure their fight. In general, when the eyes are intenfely employed upon any object,

ject, they never fhould be expofed to an oppofite
light.

If, notwithſtanding theſe precautions, or from
neglect in obſerving them, the preſent deformity
ſhould be contracted, one of the moſt approved
and fafeft remedies is contained in the following
recipe.

Take of prepared tutty, one dram ; diaphoretic
antimony, half a dram ; verdigreafe, fix grains ;
camphor, three grains : and half a dram of white
fugar-candy ; reduce them all to a powder ; and
mix it with two ounces of the fineft frefh butter,
wafhed three or four times in good white wine :—
then with about the bulk of a pea of this ointment,
rub the eye-lids, fo as part of it may enter the eye.
Let this be repeated three or four times a-day for
fome weeks, according to the obftinacy of the
complaint.

When a child is new-wakened, he ought by no
means to be expofed to a ftrong light ; for this
makes him wink clofe, which, by frequent repetition, turns into a habit, and the child winks all
his life afterwards, juft as if a grain of duft or
chaff had got into his eyes, which has a difagreeable appearance. When fuch winking is confirmed into a habit, the cure, though certainly
very difficult, is yet practicable, by attention, and
the ufe of the following fimple remedy :—namely,
in applying a fmall linen cloth, dipt in the juice
of purflane, upon the eye-lids ; repeating this two
or three times a day, and continuing the practice
for fome months.

But winking is not the only evil which is to be
feared from thus expofing a child to a ftrong light,
immediately when he awakes ; for you thus run a
confiderable rifk of weakening his fight, and frequently

quently of depriving him of it entirely. Hiftory informs us, that Dionyfius, the tyrant of Syracufe, blinded certain criminals, by confining them in a dungeon, where there was not the leaft glimpfe of light, and then expofing them fuddenly to a very ftrong one. And in the time of Charles the Fifth, Emperor of Germany, a King of Tunis was blinded by the reflection of a very fhining bafon, placed fuddenly before his eyes.

Though not immediately within our province, we cannot difmifs this article without noticing two complaints to which the eyes are fubject; and thefe are *blearednefs* and *inflammation.*

The firft is in confequence of a humour trickling down inceffantly from the eye-lids, which reddens their borders, and glues them inceffantly to one another. When this diforder is narrowly examined, it evidently appears to be occafioned by a train of fmall fuperficial ulcers, ranged almoft imperceptibly along the border of each eyelid, as well within as without; and when neglected, are very difficult of cure.

The method is, frequently to apply to the eyelids, linen cloths, dipt in a decoction of linfeed, &c. as follows :

Take a handful of the leaves of mallows and marfh-mallows ; half a handful of the flowers of colt's-foot, half an ounce of linfeed, and three drams of fennel feed ; boil thefe together in a quart of common water for a quarter of an hour, then ftrain through a clean linen-cloth, and in the ftrained liquor diffolve half a dram of the fugar of lead. Befides this, it may be neceffary to purge with fome gentle cooling phyfic, and to drink plentifully of fweetening decoctions.

An

An *ophthalmia*, or inflammation in the eye, is a
very painful and well-known complaint, arifing
fometimes from cold, and frequently from a very
acrid blood, which ftimulates the delicate veffels
of the eye, fwelling and inflaming them.

There are two forts of ophthalmia, the one,
dry, and the other moift ; but the fame method
of cure will be fuccefsful in each, which is, to
fweeten the acrimony of the blood, as well by internal as external medicines.

In the dry ophthalmia, wafh the inner part of
the eye with a collyrium, made of twelve grains
of prepared tutty, diffolved in an ounce of rofe,
and the fame quantity of plantane water, with the
addition of a fpoonful of fpirit of wine.

Take of Paul's betony, thyme, and red rofes,
each a handful ; two ftalks of mullein ; boil them
in a gallon of white wine, (or leffen the ingredients proportionably) ; and at night apply a
comprefs to the eye, dipped in this wine.

In the watery ophthalmia, bleeding, efpecially
at the neck and foot, is often neceffary ; with the
application of an eye-water made of the diftilled
waters of fennel, eye-bright, and plantane, each
an ounce, in which diffolve two grains of fugar of
lead :—if this does not fucceed, fubftitute another
more aftringent, which may be prepared of the
fame waters, with half a dram of the white troches
of Rhafis, inftead of the fugar of lead.

At the fame time drink plentifully of broth,
made of veal, chicken, crabs, and lettice.

The following *collyriums*, or *eye-waters*, are
very good to cool and repel fharp hot humours ;
they may be readily prepared ; and will more effectually

fectually anfwer their end, if affifted by the ufe of
diuretics at the fame time.

Take calamine levigated, half a dram ; rofe-
water, two ounces. Or the fame quantities of
levigated tutty, and rofe water.

Take white vitriol, fifteen grains; rofe-water,
two ounces.

Drop into the eyes, now and then, a little of
the juices of eye-bright and rue, mixed with cla-
rified honey.

With any of thefe, the eyes may be wafhed at
difcretion in all hot defluxions ; but when the
fight decays from a drynefs or a defect of the op-
tic nerve, fuch things can avail but little.

When a *poultice* is thought neceffary, you may
take half a pint of the decoction of linfeed, and
as much flower of linfeed as is fufficient to make
it of a proper confiftence. This poultice is preferable to bread and milk for fore eyes, as it will
not grow four and acid.

The following elegant compofition was communicated to the Editor of this work by a
refpectable Clergyman, who had frequently
prefcribed it with fuccefs : at the fame time here-
marked the neceffity of changing applications of
this fort, as perhaps no medicine will continue to
operate with the fame energy for any confiderable length of time ; an obfervation applicable, we
believe, in all chronic diforders.

Eye-Water which muft be made in the month of May.

Take wood-bine and violet leaves, each one
handful ; boil them in a gallon of fpring water
till reduced to two quarts ; put into the liquor a
quarter of an ounce of roch allum, with two
fpoonfuls of honey, and boil them again for a few
G   minutes ;

minutes; ftrain the liquor, and when cold, filter it; put it into bottles, and cork them very clofe

Other blemifhes of the eye, fuch as having them of different fizes; having very fierce, or what is called haggard eyes, &c. being irremediable in themfelves, come not under our plan : any more than fuch diforders as the gutta ferena, lachrymal fiftula, cataract, &c. which are within the phyfician's immediate province.

Of the CHEEKS.

The cheeks ought to be fmooth, inclining to fulnefs and rotundity, and of an equal plumpnefs. It is a defect to have them flat, hollow, full of puftules and pimples, puffed up, and unequal.

Nothing contributes more to produce the two firft faults in the cheeks, than the want of fome of the great teeth; for which reafon, one cannot be too careful of thefe teeth, efpecially in young ladies, with refpect to the cheeks. One great fault committed daily in the management of children, when they are very young, and which hurts the faces extremely, is allowing every body to kifs them. Nothing is more capable of making their cheeks flat, and of producing pimples and fuch fort of blemifhes.

Parents quietly fuffer ftrangers to kifs the tender delicate cheeks of their children, often to their difadvantage ; for this is the ordinary caufe of thofe fcabs, ring-worms, and other dangerous eruptions, which break out upon their faces. When fuch eruptions, however, make their appearance, nothing fhould be applied to repel the humour that produces them. It is better to do nothing than to do mifchief ; and a little warm
whey

whey, or barley-water, is perhaps the only thing that can be safely made use of.

When children are born with one cheek longer than the other, the deformity will sometimes disappear of its own accord ; and frequently, unless early care is taken, continue through life.— But for a preventative, let the largest cheek be washed with warm wine, in which the leaves of carduus benedictus have been boiled ; then apply a compress dipt in the same wine, and renew this once in four hours for several days ; taking care at the same time to rub the cheek gently with the fingers, to discuss the humour which swells it, and for the most part is only a simple serum ; though if permitted to remain, may grow thick.

Of the EARS.

The ears are a great ornament to the head when they are well shaped, do not exceed a certain size, are neatly placed, well bordered, and have all those little vermicular turnings and windings (which compose the external parts of this organ) in perfection.

When the *ears are too large*, the best method is to conceal a fault which cannot be corrected. One may reasonably complain of a deformity when it cannot be concealed; but to expose a deformity, as if it were a perfection, is ridiculous indeed.

Where the ear is right placed, it lies so close to the head, that you cannot put a piece of the thinnest paper between them, without moving the former. You cannot, therefore, be at too much pains to make the ears of children lie neatly. And here we must reflect on the very improper method practised in some schools, of punishing children by pulling their ears ; a practice which not only

makes

makes them grow long, broad and dangling, but is frequently productive of hardness of hearing, if not deafness itself.

Besides the other perfections above mentioned, the ears should have a very smooth skin both before and behind, without any hair being perceivable thereupon. To preserve this perfection, if they have it, and to procure it, if they have not, wash them every morning with a little vinegar and water; and if there are any hairs upon them, cut, but do not pull them out.—Heavy pendants are very apt to lengthen the ears too much.

Of the LIPS.

One of the most striking deformities in this part, is the *hare lip*, a natural fault of the formation of one of them, but most frequently of the upper, being slit perpendicularly in the middle, like that of a hare. The division is sometimes small, at other times it is double, like the letter *M*, and then termed the double hare-lip. Besides the deformity caused by this disorder, it hinders infants from sucking, and adults from speaking distinctly.

The method of cure is entirley chirurgical.

The *inside* of the lips is, in some instances, *turned outwards*. When a child is born so, this deformity does not appear an object of consequence ; for nature often corrects it of herself after a few days. All that is needful to be done in the mean time is, to bathe the lip now and then with warm wine, and to push it gently back to its natural situation. Afterwards, if nature does not complete the cure, you must apply a little of the root of spurge-olive to the nape of the neck, and let
it

it lie till it has drawn off a confiderable quantity of ferum, the abundance and acrimony of which is the common caufe of turning out the lips.

The lips, as we obferved in the firft book, are covered with a delicate fkin, which in young people becomes chapped, contracted, and very eafily cracks, efpecially during frofty weather, or in a north-wind. A fever, or an exceffive heat in the bowels, fometimes withers this fkin too, and makes it break, fo as to fall off in little fcales like bran. It alfo happens, very frequently, that when you have been touching any thing that is unclean, and put your fingers immediately afterwards to your mouth, the fkins of the lips thereby become chapped and pimpled; but if you have touched any venemous fubftance, you may not get off fo eafy.

Drinking immediately after people who have a ftrong breath, or any bad diforder is very often the caufe of pimples and puftules on the lips. The beft remedy for which is a cruft of bread applied hot to the lips.

The readieft method of curing fimple chaps, and pimples, or fcabs of the lips, is to rub them with the following pomatum, which ftands recommended in many difpenfatories, and is as good as can be made for the purpofe.

Take three ounces of the fat of veal kidney, melt it over a gentle fire, then ftrain it, and wafh it feveral times in water. Put it again upon a very flow fire, with the fame quantity of white wax, two ounces of the oil of fweet almonds, drawn by expreffion, half an ounce of fpermaceti, and a little alkanet-root, well bruifed. Melt all together gently, and ftir them well, till the alkanet has communicated its red colour to the pomatum :

then

then take it off the fire, and put it up in a galli-pot.

Or, take prepared tutty and oil of eggs, of each equal parts; mix, and apply them to the lips, after washing the latter with barley or plantane water.

Or, take hog's lard washed in rose water, half a pound; red roses, and damask roses, bruised, a quarter of a pound; knead them together, and let them lie in that state two days; then melt the hog's lard, and strain it from the roses :—add a fresh quantity of the latter, knead them in the hog's lard, and let them lie together two days as before; then gently simmer the mixture in a va-pour bath : press out the lard, and keep it for use.

Any of the foregoing will perfectly answer the intention; and compositions of this kind may be varied without end.—These salves, however, will not be of service when the lips are pimpled or scabbed from a venemous infection; or from drinking after people who have any disease. The spirit of wine, or treacle water, may then be used to greater advantage.

A practice very hurtful and dangerous to the lips of children, and which people are in general not sufficiently aware of, is giving them whistles : they are commonly daubed with paint; every body plays upon them; and there is not a servant in the house, though his lips are never so scabbed, but must use the child's whistle; to whom it is given again wet, most likely with saliva, and what may be the consequence, it is easy to guess.

Disorders in the lips are many times contracted from a cause which is never suspected, and yet is very common. We have a custom, when begin-ning

ning to write with a new-made pen, of putting the point of it to our mouth to wet it, and thereby make it draw ink more eafily. This we ought to take care of, unlefs we make the pen ourfelves, or are fure that the perfon who made it is free from difeafe ; becaufe, whoever makes a pen, always wets it, in order to try whether it will write. It is true, he wipes it afterwards ; but feldom fo well as to take off all the faliva ; and what is left of this, though it be dried, or in ever fo fmall a quantity, is a leaven which may communicate a difeafe of the lips, or any other contagious illnefs, from one perfon to another. This remark will be corroborated by reflecting on what fort of people are employed in making pens for fale.

It fometimes happens in fevers that the lips become fcabbed, which prognofticates a cure, and in this cafe do not require any application ; the beft way being to let them quite alone, and they will go off with the fever.

Thick lips are regarded by phyfiognomifts as a fign of dullnefs ; they are certainly not handfome, efpecially in the ladies. The lips are frequently rendered thick by biting them too much, in order to make them look red and pouting, and fometimes the thicknefs is the confequence of very fevere colds. It is a deformity fcarcely, if at all to be cured. Writers have recommended purgative medicines as internals, and mafticatories and blifters as external ; but as the fuccefs is very uncertain, and the trial may be dangerous, it is moft prudent of two evils to chufe the leaft.

A very *wide mouth* is juftly enough reckoned a deformity ; but it is frequently rendered more difagreeable by a habit of gaping at every object,

as

as if the perfon had never feen it before. Such
a fight is mortifying, and yet it is but too frequent
to fee people of good fenfe and judgement look
juft like idiots, only from this cuftom of gaping,
which by negligence, they have been allowed to
contract.

It muft be owned, however, that neither negligence nor ftupidity are always the caufe of this
deformity; but that there is another very common
and natural one, which is this.

In order to a free and full refpiration, the air
muft pafs and repafs conftantly through the noftrils : it is well known there is a communication
of the noftrils with the mouth, for the paffage of
the air which goes to the lungs. Now it frequently happens, that the excretory veffels of the nofe
are obftructed and choaked up in fuch a manner,
as the air cannot enter thereby into the mouth, to
purfue its courfe to the lungs : hence, either from
thefe obftructions, or fome defect in the formation
of the part, refpiration muft unavoidably be
performed by the mouth, which is thus neceffarily
kept open day and night to admit a fufficient
quantity of air. This not only obliges the perfon
to keep the mouth open, but is attended with another difagreeable confequence, that itoften forces
him to fpeak through the nofe. When thefe
defects arife from a fault in the formation of the
nofe, they are incurable. But if proceeding from
obftructions in the glands, or excretory veffels,
foftening, relaxing, deobftruent, and refolving
medicines are of fervice.—Of this number is cow's
milk mixed with the juice of beets, mallows, pellitory, wild mercury, filver-weed, and creffes,
which muft be introduced pretty warm into the
nofe as far as poffible. Or the herbs may be boiled

in

in frefh butter, and then introduced in the fame
manner.

Thefe obftructions are moftly owing to thick
humours, though they are fometimes produced by
ftoney concretions in the nofe, no bigger than a
fmall pea, and wrapped up in a membrane, which
fometimes breaks of itfelf, and lets the ftones fall
out. As it is but feldom, however, that this
membrance breaks of its own accord, the fureft
way is not to wait for it, but to ufe all the means
you can to break it gently, and without violence;
for as it adheres pretty ftrongly to the nofe, there
is danger, left in tearing it away, you fhould injure
that organ. A very good method is to introduce
the downy part of a feather into the nofe, moving
it lightly up and down; and the practice of this
method for a few weeks, efpecially in the morning
will certainly break the membrane, and of courfe
clear the obftruction. If any forenefs remains,
you may lightly touch the part with a little of the
vulnerary, or Turlington's balfam.

Of the CHIN.

Deformities of the chin in regard of fhape, are
of that clafs which can neither be prevented nor
corrected.

Women of fanguine complexions and habit,
have frequently hair growing on their chin, which
gives them a very mafculine and unfeemly appearance. Shaving, if ever fo neatly performed,
will always leave the marks of the hair percep-
tible : the only method, therefore, from which
fuccefs can be hoped, is the application of the
dulcified fpirit of falt, or fome of the liniments,
directed under the methods of extirpating fuperfluous hair.

When

When the want of beard in the other fex, proceeds from any peculiarity in the conftitution, fo
that there is not the leaft ftem of hair in the chin,
the deficiency can never be repaired by art. But
if occafioned by any accident, (which has not entirely deftroyed the roots of the hair,) as a ftraightnefs of the pores, or a want of nourifhment, a
cure may be brought about. For which purpofe,
the prefcriptions already recommended for promoting and increafing the growth of the hair may
be fuccefsfully applied.

Some people are afflicted with an involuntary,
convulfive motion of the chin, from fide to fide,
and fometimes up and down, like the motion of
eating. This deformity may be greatly relieved
by bathing; and efpecially by wafhing the part
afflicted every day with cold fpring water.

Of the SKIN, and COMPLEXION.

The fkin of the face is fubject to many accidents and deformities, which we now proceed to
examine; and firft, the effects of that very for-
midable enemy to beauty, the fmall-pox; moft
of the blemifhes caufed by which are more to be
attributed to thofe who have the management
of the diforder, than to the diforder itfelf. While
they aim at hindering the fmall-pox from thickening the fkin, and leaving pits and fcars upon it,
they generally employ means which are readier to
produce than prevent fuch effects. It is common
to apply oil of rapes, or of fweet almonds, hogs-
lard, and other greafy fubftances, as ferve rather
to fhut the pores than to open them, and likewife
make the fkin of the face very thick and coarfe.
A better method is to take a piece of very lean
mutton, boil it well, and dipping a fpunge in the
broth,

broth, gently foment the face, taking care to
repeat this several times a day, till the pustules of
the small-pox are quite ripe.

There can be no necessity for giving a caution
against picking off the eruptions, or pricking them
when the *pus* grows white, in order, as supposed, to prevent them eating through the skin. It
is, however, a constant fact that the small-pox
never leaves deeper pits, than when the pustules
have been opened, by whatever means. The
reason of this may be readily understood : when
you open the pustules, and let out the matter, you
let in the air at the same time, which immediately
dries and hardens the cavities of the pustules, and
thus prevents the flesh below from rising to fill up
the hollows. And could the face be kept from
the air from the time that the pustules fill, un-
till the patient's recovery, it would be no more
subject to injury from the disorder, than the
other parts of the body, which are never marked. A
cap might easily be contrived to answer this purpose, having its borders only at such a distance
from each other as to allow the patient to breath
freely.

The following water is of great use to prevent
pits after this disorder, clear away the scabs, allay
the itching, and remove the redness.

Dissolve an ounce and a half of salt in a pint of
mint water ;   boil them together, and dissolve the
liquor.

Of Pimples.

This deformity consists in a redness of the face,
attended with inflammatory pustules : the cause
of which is commonly attributed to an acrid, thick
blood, that swells and erodes the small vessels
which

which are diſtributed to the ſkin of the face. To clear thoſe veſſels, the maſs of blood muſt be ſweetened and diluted by proper medicines.

This is, however, a ſubject on which we would requeſt the moſt earneſt attention of our readers : —deformities of the ſkin are generally the conſequence of a diſtempered blood thrown upon it : or rather are made by a preternatural ſecretion ; for uſually ſuch diſtempers are occaſioned by the ſalts being thrown off by the cutaneous glands, which ought to be waſhed through the kidneys : ſo that inſtead of *ſweeteners,* which are uſually preſcribed, promoting the urinary diſcharges, and rectifying the ſkin by proper waſhes, is the only way to get rid of ſuch diſorders. At the end of this article, we ſhall inſert a variety of ſuch forms as ſeem beſt adapted for the purpoſe.

The application of ſuch waſhes, &c. muſt always be underſtood to be proper only, when a perſon is otherwiſe well ; becauſe any critical breakings out are by no means to be driven back, but encouraged, elſe a great deal of miſchief may be done. Of ſuch lotions too, it is to be obſerved that they are not to be uſed but for the face, and ſome particular parts ; becauſe ſo far as they are uſed, they cannot but in ſome meaſure abate the natural perſpiration, which will be attended with inconveniency. When, therefore, any thing of this kind is employed, the perſon muſt always take care that ſome other emunctory may be in readineſs to diſcharge what is leſſened by the application of the external medicine ; and that which is moſt ſuited to compenſate for what the ſkin is deficient in, is that by urine : wherefore *diuretics* are certainly the beſt auxiliaries to *coſmetics,* and

it

it is hardly fafe to ufe one without the other. For this purpofe,

Infufe four ounces of muftard feed in a quart of white-wine, and after three or four days, drink abcut a wine glafs of it every morning ; filling up the bottle every time, as long as the feed gives any ftrength.

This remedy is very eafily procured, and is not only a good diuretic, but is cordial to the nerves, attenuating pituitous, fizey blood, and diffolving its clofe contexture.

Or, boil three fpoonfuls of muftard feed in a quart of milk, take off the curd, and keep the whey for ufe.

This differs little from the above, but will be agreeable and convenient in cafes where wine would be too powerful a morning draught. About half a pint is fufficient at a time.

The *fcorbutic juices* are much commended for cooling the blood, and cleanfing the feveral ftrainers of the body, efpecially the urinary paffages ; they are moft properly ufed in the fpring, and fhould be drank about half a pint every morning for five or fix weeks.

They are prepared by taking juice of plantain, brook-lime, water creffes, and dandelion, each a pint ; forrel, lemons, and white wine, each half a pint ; let them ftand till they fettle, then decant what is clear, and add to it, of compound horfe-radifh water, and magifterial worm-water, each four ounces; fpirit of fcurvy-grafs, one ounce: and keep for ufe.

Among all the lotions invented for the affiftance of beauty, nothing perhaps can exceed the ufe of fimple *pimpernel water*, which is fo fovereign a

H   beauti-

beautifier of the complexion, as to deferve a place on every lady's toilet. It is quickly prepared, by only infufing half a handful of this herb in a quart of water, letting it ftand all night. It may be ufed a little warmifh, but never hot It is not, however, powerful enough to deftroy thofe eruptions on the face we are now treating of, for which the following applications are intended, fubject to the mode of treatment already given.

Take litharge of gold, four ounces; white wine vinegar, half a pint; digeft them together for three days, ftirring often, and then filter for ufe.

Or, take half a pound of cerus; white wine vinegar and elder-flower water, each a pint and a half; boil one point away, and let the remainder fettle fine for ufe.

Or, take camphire rubbed fine in a mortar, two drams; put upon it, by little and little at a time, one ounce of the juice of lemons; when diffolved, add white wine, one pint; or fpirit of . wine, and rofe-water, each half a pint.—This is a very fafe and good lotion for fpots and flufhings of the face, and may be ufed with equal freedom and fafety.—The mortar muft be rubbed with a few drops of oil, in order to reduce the camphire to powder.

Another, and by no means an inefficacious remedy for a pimpled face, and for preferving the fkin foft and fmooth, is, to beat a quantity of houfeleek in a marble mortar, fqueeze out the juice, and clarify it.—When wanted to ufe, pour a few drops of rectified fpirit on the juice, and it will inftantly turn milky.

A very elegant cofmetic is made by taking equal parts of gum Benjamin and ftorax, and diffolving them in a fufficient quantity of fpirit of wine.

The

The fpirit will then become a reddifh tincture, and exhale a very fragrant fmell. A few drops of it put into a glafs of water, will inftantly become milky. Many ladies ufe it, fuccefsfully, to clear the complexion, than which nothing can be more fafe or innocent.

It may not be improper to obferve, that all acid and aluminous lotions and beautifiers, are pernicious enemies to the fkin, and very foon bring on wrinkles.

Dr. Cook, of Leigh, who is as much efteemed for his philanthropy, as he is celebrated for medical knowledge, recommends the fubjoined prefcription as a fafe and excellent cofmetic lotion, " which will fet of the countenance to the beft advantage, by rendering an ordinary one beautiful, and an handfome one more fo.

" Boil two quarts of foft water on four ounces of pure quick filver, in an earthen pipkin, till half the water is wafted, then pour the water, with quick-filver and all, into a bottle to be ready for ufe :—with a fine cloth dipped into a little of this decoction, wafh the face two or three times a week in a morning, after having wafhed as ufual with frefh water.

" It gives a fine luftre to the fkin, and cleanfes it of all kinds of foulnefs, as fcurfs, infects, morphews, &c. &c. is perfectly innocent, and the beft deobftruent in phyfic. It may be drank freely as a fpecific againft worms; and againft all cutaneous eruptions.

" I remember a lady, (fays he) that had been eminent for beauty in many courts of Europe, confeffed to me that this infipid liquor was, of all innocent wafhes for the face, the beft fhe ever met with.

" The

" The fame quick-filver will ferve to boil again with the fame quantity of water, to fupply frefh lotions, as often as wanted. You muft fhake the bottle well before you ufe it."

FRECKLES.

Fair and delicate complexions are fubject to fmall reddifh fpots, called freckles; ufually caufed by the heat of the fun, and appearing chiefly on the hands, neck, and face ; for which reafon, we ought to take care of expofing children too much to its influence ; very few remedies have been found anfwerable to this blemifh, becaufe the inventors have miftaken the feat of the complaint :—— imagining it to exift in the fcarf-fkin, they have been very free in pre-fcribing corrofive waters, which make the fcarf-fkin peel off, and afterwards leave the face juft as it was : whereas thefe freckles are really upon the *cutis*, or true fkin, and become vifible from the tranfparency of the *cuticula*. They are very hard to remove ; yet much may be expected from a mixture of fpirit of wine and the oil of *Behen* [or *Ben*,] applied to the face every night with a fmall brufh :—three or four drops are fufficient at a time. But you muft avoid the air, and efpe-cially the fun-fhine during the time of ufing it.

To the fame effect are the following prepara-tions :

Take oil of tartar *per deliquium*, one ounce ; oil of fweet almonds, two drams ; rofe water, four ounces ; fhake them together for ufe.

Or, take almond-milk, (that is, an emulfion of blanched almonds,) a quarter of a pint ; fugar of
lead,

lead, ten grains; white vitriol, one fcruple; oil of tartar, two drams.

Or, take equal quantities of houfe-leek and celandine; diftil them in a fand heat, and wafh with the diftilled water.

With a foft napkin dipped in any of thefe preparations, rub the face, neck, and hands :—avoiding the fun and air.

Mr. Homberg's remedy for freckles ftands in high efteem, and is a compofition of bullock's blood and alum, nearly in this manner : — viz. To four ounces, or a quarter of a pint of bullock's blood, add two drams of alum finely powdered : let the alum precipitate, and expofe the compound three or four months to the fun in a clofe phial.

MARKS *on the* FACE.

The marks here meant are thofe which are attributed to certain longings during pregnancy : fuch as the figures of cherries, mulberries, ftrawberries, &c. or fpots of wine, milk, &c either on the face, or other parts of the body ; which are impreffed the more ftrongly in proportion to the vivacity of the mother's imagination, and the difficulty of gratifying her longing.

As to fpots of wine, milk, and fimilar ones, it is impoffible to remove them, and whoever attempts it, only defigns to impofe on you.

Such marks, or little excrefcences, as are connected to the body only by a flender ftalk, may probably be taken away ; but the ftalk muft te a very flender one indeed, or it is not advifable to touch it.

You muft tie a waxed filk thread gently about it ; next day tie it tighter : and fo proceed till

H 3   the

the excrefcence is deprived of nourifhment, when it will drop of, and nothing remain but a little fcab upon the part, which will fall away of its own accord.

The COMPLEXION *brown, pale, tawny, &c.*

When the complexion is naturally of any of thefe colours, there is no poffibility of changing it thoroughly : all that can be done, is to have recourfe to palliatives,—not to paints, which in the end produce a real deformity, but to wafhes and compofitions which are at leaft entirely harmlefs ; fuch as rofe, plantane, or pimpernel water ; water made with bran, oat-meal, peafe-meal, powder of bitter almonds; barley-water; water diftilled from fnails ; and fuch fimple preparations, from which there is nothing to fear.—To affift and improve complexional charms, where a healthful habit of body is the natural groundwork, the following very felect compofitions may prove ufeful.

A COSMETIC *for the* FACE.

1. Take a pound of levigated hartfhorn ; two pounds of rice powder ; half a pound of cerufs ; frankincenfe, gum maftic, and gum arabic, each two ounces ; diffolve the whole in a fufficient quantity of rofe-water, and frequently wafh the face with this fluid.

IMPERIAL WATER.

2. Take five quarts of brandy, or proof fpirit, in which diffolve of frankincenfe, maftic, benjamin, and gum arabic, each one ounce ; cloves and nutmegs, half an ounce ; pine-nut kernels and fweet almonds, each an ounce and a half ; to thefe add

add a few grains of muſk, or any other perfume you pleaſe ; bruiſe them very well in a marble mortar, then put them into a glaſs bottle, with the brandy, ſhaking them frequently during a week; after which let it ſettle, and decant for uſe. When applied to the face, dilute it with pimpernel, or roſe-water.

This is ſaid to take away wrinkles, render the ſkin delicate, and ſweeten the breath.

The diſtilled waters of fennel and white lillies, with a little gum maſtic, will admirably clear the complexion.

A FLUID *to clear a tanned* SKIN.

Soak unripe grapes in water ; ſprinkle them with alum and ſalt, then wrap them up in paper, and roaſt them in hot aſhes ; ſqueeze out the juice, waſh the face with it every morning, and it will ſoon remove the tan.

The oil of unripe olives, in which a ſmall quantity of gum maſtic has been diſſolved, will anſwer the ſame intention.

Another very elegant Waſh.

Take barley-water ſtrained through a fine linen cloth ; drop into it a few drops of balm of Gilead, and ſhake the bottle for ſome time, till the balſam is incorporated with the water, which will be known by its turbid, milky appearance. This greatly improves the complexion, and preſerves the bloom of youth, if only uſed once a day for a continuance. Before this fluid is uſed, the face ſhould be waſhed clean with common water.

A diſtilled

A diſtilled Water for tinging the Cheeks.

Take two quarts of white wine vinegar, three ounces of iſinglafs, two ounces of nutmegs, and ſix of honey ; diſtill with a gentle fire, and add to the diſtilled water a little red faunders, in order to colour it. Previous to the uſe of this, a lady ſhould waſh herſelf with elder-flower water, and then the cheeks will become of a lively rofeate hue, which cannot be diſtinguiſhed from the natural bloom of youth.

A Cofmetic OIL.

Take a quarter of a pint of oil of ſweet almonds freſh drawn ; one ounce of oil of tartar *per deliquium*, and a few drops of oil of rhodium ; mix them together, and uſe the compoſition for cleanſing and ſoftening the ſkin.

Oily compoſitions, (if only uſed occaſionally, and the face foon after waſhed with fome of the foregoing ſimple preparations) may be of ſervice; but laviſhly employed, they ſhut up the infenſible pores of tranfpiration, and rather injure than improve beauty.

COLD CREAM *for the* COMPLEXION.

Take virgin-wax and fpermaceti, of each a dram ; oil of ſweet almonds, two ounces ; ſpring water, an ounce and a half ; melt the wax and fpermaceti together in the oil of almonds, in a glazed earthen pipkin, over hot aſhes, or in a vapour bath ; pour the folution into a marble mortar, and ſtir it till it grow cold and quite fmooth ; then mix the water gradually, and keep ſtirring till the whole is incorporated.

This

This pomatum becomes extremely white and light by the agitation, and much refembles cream, from the fimilitude to which it has obtained its name. It is an excellent cofmetic, rendering the fkin fmooth and delicate : its fragrance may be improved by ufing rofe water or orange flower-water, inftead of fpring-water ; or with a few drops of any effence, as fancy directs.

Carmines, or Rouges for the Face.

Alkanet root ftrikes a beautiful red when mixed with oils or pomatums. A fcarlet or rofe colour-ed ribband, wetted with water or brandy, gives a beautiful bloom to the cheeks, when rubbed on them, that can hardly be diftinguifhed from the natural complexion. Many ufe only a red fponge, which tinges the cheeks with a fine carnation tint.

Or, take an equal quantity in weight of either Brazil wood fhavings, or cochineal,and roch alum; beat them together to a coarfe powder, and boil in a fufficient quantity of red wine, until two thirds of the liquor be confumed. When this decoction has ftood till cold, rub a little on the cheeks with a bit of cotton.

A very wan, fallow complexion, or that which characterizes the *green ficknefs*, is owing to a caufe that comes properly under a phyfician's confidera-tion, and is beyond our province. When the caufe is removed, the effect will ceafe of courfe.

A very frequent expofure to the open air and wind, efpecially in fummer, renders the complexion *coarfe* : there is another caufe, lefs noticed, which produces the fame effect ; namely, *fweating* : it dilates the pores exceedingly ; and thefe being dilated,

dilated, neceffarily makes the fkin appear coarfer.
By fweating we do not mean the natural perfpiration, but that which is brought on by any degree of fatigue in hot weather, or by being crowded
up in large companies, and the effects of which
is increafed by the ufe of a fan.

The complexion ought by no means to fhine,
but fhould refemble that bloom which is obfervable upon fome fruits before they are handled.
We fay the *bloom of a complexion*, but never *the
luftre* ; becaufe this does not belong to it. The
lily is white, but has no *glafs*. Yet we fay the
brightnefs of the lily. Rofes with all their brightnefs are not fhining ; yet we compliment a
complexion, by faying it is compounded of *rofes
and lilies*. In fhort, a fine fkin does not fhine
at all, although by its whitenefs it appears
bright. A fhining face is like that of a wax
baby.

To avoid this fhining, the face fhould never be
much rubbed, efpecially with coarfe cloths, nor
fhould any kind of foap be ufed in wafhing it.
Clear fpring water, or any of the fimple lotions
already defcribed, will prove the beft wafhes,
which may be rubbed dry with a foft napkin.

That the complexion fhould lofe this bloom as
age advances, is only a circumftance in the courfe
of nature ; but fome young people are not exempt
from fuch a deformity; which (when not owing to
paint) proceeds from an internal heat drying and
withering the fkin ; the fading of which may be
corrected or prevented in youthful life, by an ob-
fervance of the following rules; but 'tis childifh to
imagine there are any fecrets to preclude the effects
of old age.

1. It

1. It will be neceſſary to abſtain from tea and coffee, at leaſt not to drink much milk with them; ſhun all high ſeaſoned victuals, ſpices, ſweetmeats, wines and ſpirituous liquors, which overheat the blood, and render the ſkin wrinkled. 2. Drink plentifully of barley water, ſoups, and eat light nouriſhing food. 3. You muſt neither keep late hours, nor ſing much; and when you are dreſſing, take care no powder falls upon your face. 4. In winter, you muſt not ſit oppoſite a fire, nor too near it; and if your face is turned towards it, interpoſe a ſcreen. 5. Never expoſe yourſelf with your face uncovered to the cold air, eſpecially in froſts; nor go too ſoon near the fire after being abroad. 6. You muſt have recourſe to gentle rubbing all over the body, to preſerve or to promote a free circulation of the blood. For when the blood circulates freely, and conſequently the nouriſhing juices, which are diſtributed to the different parts of the body, neither ſtop too long, nor are hurried too quickly through the veſſels, the complexion is always freſh, provided ſuch juices are wholeſome, which may be obtained by obſerving a good regimen.— When the blood circulates well, the complexion is neceſſarily improved thereby; and always ſhews whether the health is in a good or bad ſtate.— Gentle rubbing, however, with ſoft linen, contributes very much to regulate and quicken a languid circulation, and, in conſequence of that, to enliven the complexion.

Glyſters, and gentle cathartics, when properly uſed, and not wantonly ſported with, are certainly conducive to the ſame effect.

Not as a cure, but as a preventative of wrinkles, the ſubjoined preparations appear to have ſome efficacy.

1. How

1ſt. Heat an iron ſhovel red hot, throw on it ſome powder of myrrh, and receive the ſmoak on your face, covering your head with a napkin to prevent its being diſſipated. Repeat this operation three times. Heat the ſhovel again, and pour on it a mouthful of white wine. Receive the vapour of the wine alſo on your face, repeating it three times. Continue this practice every night and morning, as long as you ſhall find occaſion.

2d. Take juice of white lily roots, and fine honey, each two ounces; white wax melted, one ounce; incorporate the whole together, and make a pomatum, which muſt be applied every night, and not wiped off till the next morning.

Having finiſhed our remarks on thoſe parts of the face which are moſt expoſed to view, we come next to treat of ſuch as preſent themſelves on opening the mouth, viz. the gums, teeth, and tongue, which cloſes our review of the head, or upper cavity of the human body.

Of the GUMS.

Thoſe gums which are red, firm, ſmooth, neither too thick nor too thin, and have the teeth neatly joined within them, are a great ornament, provided that every thing about the teeth be proportionable and correſponding.

The livid colour of the gums generally proceeds from the blood ſtagnating there, which may be prevented or corrected by rubbing them carefully every morning with a linen cloth, a little rough, and picking them from time to time, but very gently, with the point of a gold, ſilver, or ivory tooth-pick, but yet ſo as to make them bleed;
and

and taking care not to pick it where the teeth are joined to the gum.—Some writers have told us, that eating of leeks and onions is hurtful to the gums.

Excrefcences will fometimes appear upon the gums, connected to them by a little flender ftalk; a circumftance of no danger, but often a blemifh, by making the lips protrude forward in a difagree-able manner, and affecting the pronunciation a little. This excrefcence may eafily be taken off, by tying a thread of filk pretty tight round it, and drawing it ftill tighter every day for a few days, when it will drop off for want of nourifhment; and you may touch the gum with a little vul-nerary balfam.

An inflammation of the gums, being a confe-quence of the inflammatory tooth-ach, will be treated in its proper place.

As moft other blemifhes or deformities of the gums, as being pale, flaccid, uneven, fretted, &c. may be attributed to the fcurvy in that part, we fhall avoid all nice diftinctions, and only confider that diforder in general,

One certain fymptom of the fcurvy is, the gums being liable to bleed on the flighteft touch:—another is a continual difcharge of matter from about the edges, juft where they join the teeth, but without any appearance of blood; and a third (which may likewife have a temporary exiftence from other caufes, as venereal infections, ulcera-tions of the lungs, and particularly negligence in cleaning the teeth) is an offenfive breath, fre-quently unknown to the perfon himfelf. Thefe fymptoms are fometimes all experienced together, and often are found independent of each other. The teeth, in this diforder, are in fome perfons

I   covered

covered with a tartareous matter, and in others remarkably clean. In procefs of time, they become quite loofe; and when the diftemper is fo far advanced, 'tis with difficulty that any thing can be done to prevent them all dropping out, one after another, though perfectly found. Not that the gums always recede from the teeth; for they will fometimes preferve an external appearance of foundnefs, even when the fcurvy has totally deftroyed the bony focket, and all communication between the tooth and gum.

The fcurvy in the gums feldom extends beyond that part, and is certainly very different from, as it frequently is found independent of the leaft degree of the fcurvy in the body, and without any connection with it: the former having been perfectly cured, when the latter has not had the fmalleft relief. Nor is any advantage to be expected from the ufe of internal medicine.

The firft ftep towards a cure, is to have the teeth well cleaned, and all the tartareous matter that is lodged under the edges of the gums, carefully removed, by a fkilful dentift: when the complaint is not of long continuance, this operation will prevent its farther progrefs: tho' it is frequently fo long neglected, as to require the application of the lancet; and when the gums are much thickened, it even becomes neceffary that confiderable portions of them fhould be taken off.

When the diforder is once put a ftop to, it may be prevented in future by a proper attention to the cleanlinefs of the teeth, and ufing fome of the following lotions occafionally to the gums; while a neglect of this will often caufe a relapfe;— Wafhing and brufhing the gums produce the fame effect

effect on them, as air and exercise upon the body; giving vigour and firmnefs, promoting the circulation, and enlivening the tone of both.

To ftrengthen and preferve the Gums.

Diffolve an ounce of myrrh (finely powdered) as much as poffible, in a pint of red wine; decant it off, and wafh the mouth every night and morning

To ftrengthen the Gums, and make them grow clofe to the Enamel.

To two fpoonfuls of the beft white honey, add an ounce of myrrh, and a little green fage, both finely powdered; mix them well together, and rub the teeth and gums with a little of this balfam every night, at going to reft.

An Infufion for the Gums.

Take two drams of cinnamon finely powdered ; half a dram of cloves in fine powder ; and half an ounce of roch alium ; pour upon them three quarts of boiling water, when cold, add fix ounces of plantane water, half an ounce of orange-flower (or any other fcented) water ; a quarter of an ounce of effence of lemon, or of bergamot ; and three quarters of a pint of rectified fpirit of wine, or good brandy ; let the whole ftand in digeftion for a few days, then decant for ufe.

An ounce of Peruvian bark, grofsly powdered, infufed in half a pint of brandy, and diluted with an equal quantity of rofe water, is efteemed very ferviceable in preferving the gums.

Oak leaves boiled in fpring water, with a few diops of fpirit of fulphur added to the decoction, afford a very ufeful gargle for the mouth and gums.

When

When the teeth have been once properly cleaned, and such necessary operations performed, as the judgement of a sensible operator will dictate, the gums may be easily kept in tolerable condition afterwards by the use of any of the foregoing preparations, constantly and daily used; but it is from perseverance alone that any benefit may be expected. Even the application of cold water daily to the gums, rubbing them well with a little brush, or your finger, will equally preserve them from disorder, and the teeth from decay. Those who pay a constant attention to this point, have in general few decayed teeth, and even when a decay takes place, it advances more slowly, and with much less pain.

An *offensive breath* is a constant attendant upon the scurvy in the gums, but may also proceed from putrified matter lodged in hollow teeth; or from other causes as above-mentioned; in any case, it may at least be disguised, if not greatly remedied, by gargling the mouth frequently with the following water.

Take fresh gathered (if conveniently procured, if not, take dry'd) leaves of sage, angelica, wormwood, savory, fennel, and spiked mint, hyssop, balm, sweet basil, rue, thyme, marjoram, rosemary, origanum, calamint, and wild thyme, each four ounces, the same quantity of lavender flowers, cut them small, pour upon them one gallon of good brandy, or spirit of wine, and let them stand in a warm situation for a week or thereabouts; then decant for use.

To half a wine glass of this tincture, add the same quantity of rose water, or any other distilled water you fancy, gargle the mouth well (rubbing the

the gums with your finger) with about half of 't, and rince the mouth with the remainder.

If half or a whole glafs of this tincture, diluted as before, be drank every morning, after the above operation, it will cherifh the lungs, enliven the heart, fortify the ftomach, and cleanfe them of every impurity that may affect the breath. It is likewife much fuperior to preparations from caftern aromatics and perfumes, whofe very powerful fcent only difcovers what their ufe is defigned to conceal.

Of the latter fort, however, the following ftands in high efteem.

Take cinnamon, two ounces; cloves, fix drams; Florentine orrice root, nutmeg, and mace, each one dram; water crefles, fix ounces; frefh lemon peel, an ounce and a haif; red rofe leaves, an ounce; fcurvy grafs, half a pound; mufk and ambergreafe, each half a fcruple; bruife the aromatics and perfumes, cut the fpices, and macerate the whole in a quart of fpirit of wine, or French brandy, during eight-and-forty hours; then decant it into feveral glafs phials, fo that having a fmall quantity only in ufe at a time, the fragrant effence may be prevented from evaporating. When ufed, let it be diluted with any diftilled water.

As a more fimple remedy, chew about the quantity of a fmall nut of gum myrrh, at night going to bed.

Or, chew every night and morning a clove; or a piece of Florentine orrice root, about the fize of a bean.

The Eaftern nations frequently chew boiled Chio turpentine, or gum maftick, which is faid to give health and firmnefs to the gums, make the

teeth

teeth beautifully white, and procure a fweet breath.

People who are accuftomed to thefe daily ablutions of the teeth and gums, are much lefs liable to the infection of malignant, epidemic diforders, than when the gums are in a ftate of putrefaction, and the teeth covered with fordes. Befides, the air in paffing through the mouth into the lungs, muft of courfe be contaminated, and impregnated with the putridity of the gums, or of matter in, or between the teeth ; which will doubtlefs produce fome, and increafe almoft any diforder.

Of the Teeth.

To preferve the teeth in order, and in any degree of beauty, requires lefs trouble than perfeverance. Five minutes labour every morning, and the examination by a dentift once in a month, or perhaps in a quarter of a year, is amply fufficient. Indeed, to produce a fet of fine, regular teeth, they fhould be taken under management from their very firft appearance, and every affiftance given to make them cut eafy, and pufh out regular; otherwife they have lefs chance to be well fhaped, well ranged, and make a beautiful appearance.—The firft teeth prepare fockets for thofe which are to fucceed them; and upon the right difpofition of thefe fockets will the regularity and beauty of the fecond fet of teeth depend.

The breeding and cutting of the teeth often prove fatal to infants, at all times is attended with violent pains, and frequently with convulfions and fevers. Loofenefs, if not fevere, is rather a favourable fymptom. Diluting liquors, as milk and water, balm tea, &c. fhould be plentifully adminiftered, administered, but by no means too warm. The appearance of the teeth are usually foretold by a small white circle surrouding that part of the gum, and describing the fize of the future tooth; at this time it will be necessary to rub the gums with a little fine honey mixed with liquorice powder; which frequently prevents convulsions; the white shank of a boiled asparagus, or the rib of a large lettice leaf, is often successfully employed to rub the gums with.

The difficulties and dangers which attend teething may frequently be obviated, and considerably lessened, by attending to a few plain, general rules.- To keep the body open by cooling and corrective medicines;—to guard against any violent loosenesses by a proper change of physic;—to supply the want of immediate operation by gentle clysters or vomits; and taking care that the food be very light, (if the child is weaned) as chicken broth, beef tea, or palatable flops, which are preferable to flesh meals.

For this purpose, rhubarb; with magnesia, in case of costiveness; or with prepared crabs-claws, in case of too great a degree of loofenefs; clyfters made with mutton or chicken broth,—common salt, coarse sugar, and sweet oil,—adapting the quantity to the age of the child.

When the efforts of nature, assisted by this treatment, are insufficient to burst the gum, and any alarming symptoms of inflammation or convulsions appear, the lancet should be applied.

When the first teeth are compleated, little attention is required, except to examine the double teeth occasionally; and, as they are most subject to decay, to file or stop them, as may be required.

From

From the earlieſt infancy, children ſhould be taught to waſh their teeth and gums every morning and evening with cold water, and continue this practice through life.

About ſix or ſeven years of age, they begin to ſhed theſe firſt teeth, and new ones ſucceed, the preſervation and management of which demand our vigilant attention.

Even, regular teeth contribute ſo much to the beauty of the human countenance, that without their aid, the viſage would appear deformed, and the harmony of the fineſt features be incomplete. Irregularity might be often prevented by a timely removal of the firſt ſet of teeth, whenever they appear crooked, projecting forward, inclining inwards, or otherwiſe tending to deformity, as they give the ſhape to the bony ſocket for thoſe which are to follow: and hence diſtort the mouth, and affect the ſhape of the whole face.

There is another deformity which ſeems cauſed by inattention to the teeth in early life; namely, when the teeth of the under jaw project forward beyond thoſe of the upper, and incloſe them; the contrary to which being the natural ſituation. This being *under-jawed,* not only renders the front teeth uſeleſs in both jaws in eating, but makes the under one grow conſiderably longer than it otherwiſe would.—The correction, or prevention of this deformity, muſt be under the management of a ſurgeon, as it requires manual operation.

The teeth ſhould be often examined from ten or twelve years of age, to obſerve their decay, and make the neceſſary proviſion againſt it: to prevent the caries from reaching the nerve; and alſo to remove all tartareous accumulations which may

have

have adhered to them, and which, by a ſkilful and
honeſt operator, may be taken off without the
leaſt injury to the ſofteſt enamel.

Thoſe concretions about the teeth and gums,
which are called the tartar of the teeth, proceed
from a hurtful nutriment ; partly from the
ſaliva, impregnated with the excrementitious
juice of the gums, which by continually moiſtening the teeth, gradually adds theſe tartareous par-
ticles to them. This tartar, in conſequence of its
acrimony, imperceptibly conſumes the ſubſtance
of the teeth, produces blackneſs, and frequently a
caries or rottenneſs : It evidently conſiſts of an
alkaline earth, by inſtantly reſolving when rubbed
with ſpirit of ſalt.

The outward ſubſtance, or enamel of the teeth,
is of a very hard contexture, almoſt approaching
to ſtone, though diſſolvable in an acid menſtruum.
The interior bone is eaſily diſſolved and conſumed.
It is the part principally affected in a caries or
rottenneſs ; for the enamel is ſeldom ſeen totally,
but only partially conſumed. And though acid
ſpirits, ſuch as the ſpirit of ſalt, ſpirit of vitriol,
&c. diſſolves the tartareous ſubſtance on the teeth,
yet too frequent, too long, or any injudicious application thereof, will deſtroy the tooth itſelf. The
foundeſt human tooth, if put into a ſolution of
ſpirit of vitriol, in proportion of ſixty grains to
one ounce of water, for the ſpace of fourteen or
fifteen days, would entirely loſe its enamel. The
effect of ſuch a preparation, therefore, when made
uſe of to clean the teeth, and frequently, perhaps
daily, applied, may be deduced from this experiment.

Acids of every denomination are unfriendly to
the teeth : whether ſpirit of ſalt, vitriolic ſpirit,

tartar of vitriol in its acid ftate, cream of tartar, or alum, burnt or unburnt. Nor are thefe the only preparations from which danger is to be apprehended : powder of coral, cuttle fifh bone, pumice-ftone, and fimilar fubftances, when frequently ufed, deftroy the enamel not lefs, though in a different manner, than the foregoing acids. The one diffolves; the other, by its afperities, acts like a file, and rubs it off. This feems to exclude all the generally received preparations for the teeth, and with great juftice; but we hope to offer others in their place, which will equally anfwer every good intention, without caufing the leaft difagreeable confequence.

Moft people may obferve, that, however clean their teeth are on going to bed at night, yet on paffing a finger over them next morning, they will be found covered with a thin, flimy fubftance, refembling thin pafte, of different colours and confiftence in different conftitutions : this fubftance, which feems the refiduum of the faliva, united with an excrementitious juice from the gums, indurates about the teeth, and acquires a degree of hardnefs little inferior to themfelves. A compofition, therefore, which will abforb this mucous fubftance, prevent it from adhering to the teeth, and preferve their natural colour, is the beft tooth-powder that can be made ufe of. That artificial whitenefs which is caufed by ufing alum, and fimilar fubftances, is a certain indication of their approaching decay, which is foon after more fenfibly announced by chillnefs and pain.

When the teeth are once perfectly freed from tartar, (which often lurks under the gums, unknown to one's felf,) the frequent ufe of the following powder will preferve them for years.

Reftorative

Reſtorative Powder for the Teeth and Gums.

Take French, or Armenian bole, one ounce ; dragon's blood and myrrh, each half an ounce ; maſtick, a dram and a half; cinnamon and cloves, each half a dram ; reduce them into a very fine powder; and with your finger dipped therein, rub the teeth and gums well two or three times a week, rincing the mouth afterwards with cold water. This comforts and ſtrengthens the gums, abſorbs all that acrimonious ſlime ' and foulneſs, which would accumulate to the deſtruction of the teeth, and has this peculiar property, that it *never can do them an injury.*

To ſuch as are deſirous of preparations that will more ſpeedily whiten the teeth, we ſhall communicate a few receipts for that purpoſe.

Take myrrh, roch alum, dragon's blood, and cream of tartar, each one ounce ; muſk two grains: make them into a fine powder.

The author of this recipe is ſo honeſt as to add, " that, tho' ſimple, it is an efficacious dentifrice : yet nothing of the kind ſhould be applied too frequently to the teeth, for fear of hurting the enamel."

If the teeth and gums are rubbed with a piece of clean rag, dipped in vinegar of ſquills, it will not only whiten, but faſten the roots of the teeth, and correct an offenſive breath.

When the enamel of the teeth is waſted, either by a ſcorbutic humour, or any external cauſe ; the tooth cannot long remain ſound, and muſt therefore be cleaned with great caution. For which purpoſe, the beſt inſtrument is a piece of wood, like a butcher's ſcewer, made ſoft at the end, and either uſed alone or dipped in the reſtorative powder recommended above.

But

But the roots of some particular plants, especially fibrous and woody ones, are best formed into little brushes for cleaning the teeth, and probably have been substituted in the room of common tooth-brushes, on account of their being softer to the gums, and more conveniently used.

Lucern and liquorice roots are generally preferred. They may be deprived of their juicy parts by boiling them several times in a large quantity of fresh water : they should be chosen of two year's growth, and about the thickness of one's little finger ; such as are thicker, worm-eaten, or unsound, being rejected. They are to be cut into pieces about six inches long; and, as we have observed, boiled in water, till all the juicy parts are extracted, then taken out and left to drain :— after this, each of the roots is to be slit with a penknife into the form of a little brush, and the roots slowly dried, to prevent their splitting. They may be dyed red by infusing them in the following liquid.

Take Brazil wood rasped, four ounces ; cochineal bruised, three drams ; roch-allum half an ounce ; water, four pints ; put them into a proper vessel, boil till one half of the liquor is consumed, and strain the decoction through a piece of linen cloth.

Let the roots remain twenty-four hours in this infusion, then take them out, dry them slowly, and let them be varnished with two or three coats of a strong mucilage of gum tragacanth, each being suffered to dry before another is laid on. The whole is afterwards repeatedly anointed with Fryar's, or Turlington's balsam, in order to form a varnish less susceptible of moisture.

Marsh-

Marſh-mallow roots are prepared in an eaſier manner; but, on account of the mucilage they contain, they become very brittle when dry. Such as are large and very even are made choice of, and raſped with a knife to remove the outer bark. They are dyed and varniſhed in the ſame manner as the others; but from the loſs of their mucilage, diminiſh conſiderably in thickneſs during the time they ſtand in fuſion.

They are uſed in a ſimilar manner with tooth-bruſhes; by moiſtening one of the ends with a little water, and having dipped it in the dentifrice you make uſe of, rub the teeth well therewith.

The large double teeth, (two on each ſide next the *dentes ſapientiæ*) are often diſcovered, even at their firſt appearance, to have ſeveral ſmall holes; and as theſe teeth are not ſucceeded by any others, care ſhould be taken, as early as poſſible, to ſtop the holes up, otherwiſe they daily enlarge, break into one, and become attended with much pain.

When the hollows of decayed teeth are filled up, whether with gold or other materials, the perſon ſhould avoid cracking nuts, or ſqueezing any hard ſubſtance between them, as that will not only cauſe the ſtopping to come out, but frequently break even ſound teeth.

Of the Tooth-Ach.

There are ſo very few perſons who have not, at ſome period of their life, experienced this diſorder, that there is no need to deſcribe it: It proceeds from a variety of cauſes, but, perhaps, from no one more frequently than neglect of cleanlineſs; rottenneſs of the teeth is only a ſecondary cauſe, or a conſequence of the former; and it is certain

K   tha

that no inftances are to be met with of diforders *originating* in the *internal part* of a found tooth, which, however, is commonly the feat of complaint; always, indeed, in decayed teeth, probably occafioned by the air entering the decayed part, and affecting the blood-veflels, or nervous membranes.

There is a cavity very confpicuous in the middle of all the teeth, and very confiderable in the bafe, or that part which appears without the gums: in this cavity there is always found a mucous, membranaceous fubftance, in the form of an oblong bladder, compofed of highly flender blood-veflels, nervous membranes, and a certain glutinous fubftance : this alfo reaches to the very extremities of the teeth, where its membranes being more contracted, it appears fomewhat harder and redder. This matter may be commodioufly feen by the naked eye, in what is called the *fweet tooth* in calves : it difcovers fome traces of blood in its furface, by a reddifh colour; and when the matter is compreffed, it actually difcharges blood ; as it will alfo do in the human teeth on application of the actual cautery, or a fmall wire made hot. This is the feat of the common tooth-ach ; which is occafioned either by the external air, the preffure of the food in eating, or being touched by any fubftance very hard, very hot, or or very cold.

Before the decay becomes confiderable, pain may be prevented by filling up the vacancy with gold, filver, gold-beater's lead, or fome proper compofition. The decay may fometimes be ftopped by properly filing the teeth in queftion. But fuch operations require the affiftance of a careful dentift.

Remedies

Remedies for this complaint are without number. When the diforder is flight, it may frequently be alleviated by applying a bit of cotton, dipped in oil of cloves, or Turlington's balfam, to the hollow part, and, if frequently repeated, will oftimes effect a cure. Tincture of laudanum or opium may alfo be ufed for the fame purpofe.

Cauterizing behind the ear ; or an actual cautery applied to the decayed tooth, relieves and often cures; and perhaps the latter operation might be beft performed by the patient himfelf, if he has refolution for the purpofe, by applying a fmall hot wire to the offending part of the tooth.

When the extirpation of tartar from under the gums has long been neglected, it frequently corrodes that part of the tooth where the enamel ends; and brings on a difagreeable fenfation, which is generally heightened by eating acids, fruit, fweetmeats, &c. The fame complaint is frequently brought on by ufing hard, cutting fubftances, under the name of tooth-powders ; it may be prevented from going further by the ufe of the reftorative powder before recommended. Indeed the very clofe adhefion of the tartareous matter will produce a pain not eafily diftinguifhable from the common tooth-ach, but which always fubfides on removing the caufe.

Severe colds, violent exercife, fitting up late, or exceffive drinking, will bring on a tooth-ach of different kind f om the foregoing, being attended with violent head-ach, fwelling of the cheeks, and an inflammation of the gums, that frequently fuppurates. It moftly begins with a gnawing pain about the roots, efpecially of the double teeth,

K 2

the

the pulfe quickens, and a fever enfues, with increafed pain, for three or four days, till the inflammation arrives to its height, the difcharge whereof commonly gives relief.

Slight electrical fhocks, or rather fparks drawn from the tooth ; bleeding, efpecially by leeches applied near the feat of the complaint ; and gentle evacuations by ftool, will be found of great fervice. Sometimes a flannel cloth foaked in a ftrong decoction of camomile, applied warm as it can be borne, and repeated quickly, will very much alleviate the complaint.

A blifter behind the ear, when the pain is extremely violent, may be applied with advantage ; and fmoking either common or herb tobacco (the latter is leaft weakening to the ftomach) will afford a temporary relief ; though fuch means cannot totally remove the diforder, which is too deeply rooted to be eradicated by thefe fuperficial remedies.

When bleeding and other applications fail, let the patient take an ounce of nitre divided into fixteen dofes ; abftaining from flefh-meat, wine, and hot liquors.

Generally, as the inflammation increafes, the feverity of the pain declines ; and in fome, tho' few cafes, the inflammation will be very confiderable without any pain whatever. Should the diforder be fo violent as to endanger the palate of the mouth, by the fecret lodgement of any acrimonious matter, the cafe becomes highly alarming, and requires the choiceft medical affiftance.

Opiates may be advantageoufly adminiftered, and often afford confiderable relief, when applied as a plaifter fo as to cover the affected part.

The

The infl ammatory tooth-ach is the common, and perhaps the only origin of gum-boils, a morbid affection of the gums, fo called ; and one of the very few caufes which can render it neceffary to extract a tooth.

It fhould be obferved, that during the inflammation, it will be very improper to attempt extracting the painful tooth ; the roots being at that time fo tightly wedged in their fockets, as to render it liable to be broken in the operation; without faying any thing of the very excruciating pain it caufes at this time.

There is a third tooth-ach, which feems to be a particular fort of rheumatifm ; for we may often obferve pains of the joints and fhoulders tranflated to one fide of the head, the teeth of which they attack in a moft violent manner. On the contrary, pains of the head and teeth are obferved frequently to change their feats, and fall upon the fhoulders and arms. As a rheumatifm is brought on by an intemperate, or fudden change of air, fo a tooth-ach of this clafs is generally excited by a fudden removal from a warm to a cold air; or by the fudden changes of heat and cold in the fpring and autumn. Rheumatifms are more incident to women than men, fo alfo are tooth-achs, though they generally prove far more fevere in the latter than in the former. Befides, it is confirmed by experience, that fuch as are fubject to rheumatic and gouty complaints, are much lefs afflicted with this tooth-ach : hence it fhould follow, that the regimen and method of cure fhould be fimilar with thofe diforders.

As in rheumatifms and gouts, fo in this tooth-ach, thofe who have been once afflicted are eafily, and by every flight caufe, fubjected to frefh attacks of the diforder, on account of the weaknefs left

K 2   behind.

behind. Thefe pains, too, are fometimes periodical ; often continue a week or ten days, almoft
without intermiffion, and then fubfide entirely for
a fortnight, or longer, when they return as b:-
fore.

This diforder is ufually treated as nervous or
rheumatic ; and when the pain has been fo intenfely violent as to refift the force, and elude the
efficacy of all other medicines, Hoffman tells us,
that he has obferved a moft fingular and unex-
pected relief afforded by the following pills invented by himfelf.

Take of the *pilulæ aleophanginæ*, one dram ;
of the *pilulæ de ftyrace* half a dram ; and of the
extract of faffron fix grains; mix them into a mafs,
of which form fixty pills ; fix or eight of them are
to be given for a dofe.

Extraction of the tooth is the laft remedy that
can be propofed, when the particular one can be
difcovered. But it muft be obferved, that there
are rheumatic and nervous pains in the head, entirely unconnected with, and independant of the
teeth ; and from which, were all the teeth in the
head drawn out, the patient would not find the
fmalleft relief. And, indeed, thofe who fuffer
their teeth to be pulled out when firm and found,
pay very little regard to their own welfare: for tooth
drawing is not only a painful operation, but is
often attended with bad accidents, and even fometimes endangers the patient's life. Æfculapius,
who, we are told, invented the art, had a pair of *leaden pullicans* hung up in a temple dedicated to him,
very properly fignifying, that no teeth were fit to
be pulled out, but fuch as could be removed with
a leaden forceps ; that is, fuch as were loofe and
ready to fall out of themfelves.

Tooth-

Tooth-drawing, however wrong, injudicioufly, or wantonly performed in fome cafes, is certainly right and neceffary in others. 1. In children, for removing the firft fet of teeth, which when left too long in their fockets, difplace the new ones, and turn them awry. 2. In infants it is alfo neceffary to draw fuch teeth as grow out of the palate, or out of improper parts of the mouth, and are fo placed as to impede fucking or fpeaking. 3. In fome certain cafes of the tooth-ach, as a laft refort, when medicines have been of no avail. 4. Such teeth, as by their irregular pofition and figure, lacerate the gums and lips, and cannot be brought into fhape by the file.

And laftly, it is fometimes neceffary to draw a tooth for the curing a fiftula, or ulceration of the gums near the roots of the teeth.

One argument that might diffuade people from flying to this operation on every trifling caufe, is the very great injury the face fuftains in its beauty. A diminution takes place, both in length and breadth ; the cheeks in particular fall in and look lanky ; and the whole vifage appears no larger than that of a child.

We fhall conclude this article with enumerating a few particulars, a want of attention to which is often of prejudice not only to people's teeth, but frequently even to health itfelf.

1. Expofing themfelves to catch cold, by walking late abroad, fleeping with the head too thinly covered, or ftanding too long oppofite to a gate , or window, half open—which occafion a flux of humours to fall on the teeth, creating the tooth-ach, fwelling of the cheeks, &c.

2. Neglect-

2. Neglecting to keep the arms and legs sufficiently warm, is often attended with as great prejudice to the teeth, as suffering cold in the head from the same neglect.

3. Not taking proper care of the head, by combing it frequently : which negligence prevents this part from perspiring so freely as it ought, whence the superfluous humour falls down upon the teeth and gives birth to several complaints.

4. Eating or drinking things that are too hot, as coffee, tea,&c. or holding hot spirituous liquors, caustic oils, and spices in the mouth for the toothach, which give a temporary ease, but lay the foundation of future pains.

5. Nothing is more apt to loosen the teeth, and rub off the enamel, than picking them with a quill-tooth-pick ; for that part of the quill which the tooth-pick is made of, is a very hard elastic substance, and very sharp ; by being passed backwards and forwards between the teeth, it acts almost as a file, wears the cortical part, and at last totally destroys it. And we may very readily observe, that the teeth generally grow carious first at the sides, where the tooth-pick is most employed. Gold and silver are not so elastic as the point of a quill, nor do the least injury by friction against the teeth. Ivory finely polished, and wrought into tooth-picks, are not injurious ; but mastic wood or bistort root are much superior, as by their astringent quality they strengthen and preserve the gums.

6. Eating sweetmeats, which by their viscidity stick close to the teeth, and corrode them ; chewing things that are too hard, or cracking the stones, of fruit or nuts, &c. eating green fruit, pickles,

p̓ickles, &c. which fret the gums; chewing food that is tough and fibrous, as cod and ſtock-fiſh, neglecting to waſh the mouth after eating, eſpecially any of the foods juſt mentioned ; with the frequent uſe of high ſeaſoned diſhes.

There are ſome people whoſe teeth are naturally black, in which caſe no art whatever can render them beautiful : the moſt that we profeſs is, to preſerve beauty where it exiſts, or to reſtore it when ſuffering by negligence : thoſe who do more deſign to prey upon the credulity of the world.

The loſs of teeth is frequently ſupplied by art, and ſometimes with ſucceſs ; though it is but fair to add, that the ſucceſs depends more upon chance, than any principles of art : and tranſplanted teeth have often been obliged to be removed, to prevent worſe conſequences. The conditions requiſite for this operation, will ſhew the little confidence that ought to be placed in its ſucceeding : and the decayed tooth muſt be one of thoſe in the front of the mouth, the operation rarely, if ever, anſwering with the double teeth, particularly the large ones.

When the decayed tooth is extracted, the ſubſtituted one muſt be immediately taken out of the perſon's mouth who is willing to loſe it; it muſt be quite ſound, of the ſame length, breadth, and thickneſs, and taken from the correſponding part of the jaw with the decayed tooth : this reſemblance, however, is only to be found among the fore-teeth. The neck of the *extracted* tooth, and what remains of its roots, ſhould be perfectly ſound.—The perſon from whom the tooth is taken to be tranſplanted, ſhould be between the age of twelve and fifteen, healthy, and of the ſame

ſex

fex with the party who is to undergo the operation. As foon as fixed, the tooth muſt be
fecured to the neighbouring ones, by liga-
tures of gold wire, filk, &c. No uſe muſt be
made of it for ſeveral days, till the gum grows to
the root of the tooth. And the attendance of a
phyſician is frequently neceſſary to regulate the
conſequent fever, which is ſometimes conſiderable.
This operation is difficult,—no artiſt can honeſtly
pretend to aſſert its ſucceſs; and the conſequence
is ſometimes diſagreeable.

Deficiencies of the teeth are better, perhaps,
ſupplied by artificial ones, whether ſingle or in
whole fets ; by the uſe of which the proportion
of the face is preſerved, and even maſtication may
be performed with eaſe and comfort.

The fame attention to cleanlineſs is requiſite
in the artificial as in natural teeth ; as they are
equally liable to decay, and in ſimilar caſes to
create an offenfive breath.

Of the Tongue.

To finiſh this book, it remains to examine ſome
of the chief defects of the tongue and voice with
reſpect to the ſpeech ; which are chiefly dumbneſs, loſs of voice, an effeminate voice in men,
and a maſculine one in women ; lifping, ſtam-
mering, and a difficulty of pronouncing certain
letters.

Of all the defects of our bodily organs, there is
ſcarce any one more mortifying than *dumbneſs*, as
hindering us from expreſſing our thoughts, and
reducing us to the ſad neceſſity of explaining them
by ſigns and grimaces. Dumbneſs may proceed
from various cauſes; as, a bad conformation of
the tongue, a palſey, or too great humidity of
it;

it ; blood ſtagnated under the tongue, or a
natural deafneſs.

Dumbneſs from a miſhapen or faulty tongue
is inde'd incurable : but as that cauſe cannot be
diſtinguiſhed from the other two, of a palſey, or
a too great humidity of the tongue, the practice
proper for the latter can do no injury in the former caſe.

When a palſey occaſions, or is only the ſuppoſed
cauſe of this complaint, you ought to have
recourſe to medical aſſiſtance ; the uſe of vine-
leaves, freſh ſqueezed, and uſed by way of drink,
(to the quantity of two ounces every day) made
palatable with a little ſugar, has been ſuccefsful,
after the ineffectual trial of almoſt every other medicine. Strong efforts to ſpeak are alſo of the
utmoſt conſequence, and on which medical writers
greatly inſiſt, corroborating its efficacy by many
hiſtorical relations.

The ſtory of *Atys*, ſon of Crœſus, king of Ly-
dia, is ſo powerful an example, and ſo well au-
thenticated by hiſtory, that we cannot forbear
noticing it : He was dumb even from his birth,
which renders the caſe ſtill more remarkable. In
the battle againſt Cyrus, ſeeing a ſoldier with an
uplifted ſcymetar ready to ſtrike off his father's
head, the emotion which ſo terrible a ſpectacle
raiſed in him, made him cry out with an effort as
violent as it was natural.—*Stop, ſoldier! kill not
my father!*—He retained his ſpeech ever afterwards.

A ſimilar inſtance is recorded by an eminent
medical writer : * A peaſant benig extremely
thirſty, after working very hard in a hot ſummer's
day, took a draught of cold water, and became
dumb immediately after ; the water occaſioning
a palſey

a palfey of the tongue. He paſſed a whole year in this melancholy ſituation without hopes of recovery: but one day, as he was carrying a heavy burthen upon his ſhoulders, compoſed of ſeveral parcels, he fell down with them in ſuch a manner that he broke his leg. The pain occaſioned by the hurt, obliged him inſtantly to make a ſtrong effort to call for help, which raiſed ſo violent a motion in the muſcles of his tongue, that they recovered their action ; and the man was immediately reſtored to his ſpeech.

Too great humidity of the tongue, though not attended with a palfey, may produce a dumbneſs, that is uſually cured of courſe by the tongue's becoming drier, as the perſon advances in years. There is a well-known inſtance of this in Maximilian, ſon of the Emperor Frederick the third, who was nine years of age before he could ſpeak; and at the end of this period, which is the time when the ſuperabundant humours of childhood begin to be dried up, he got the uſe of his tongue ſo freely as to be able to ſpeak with eaſe, and even eloquence. Many inſtances in private life might be adduced of children continuing dumb for ſome years, and yet recovering or attaining the uſe of ſpeech. Dumbneſs from this cauſe is frequently periodical.

When dumbneſs proceeds from a ſtrangulation of the veſſels under the tongue, the moſt certain method of curing it is by bleeding in that part.

In order to cure the want of ſpeech, when occaſioned by deafneſs, it is plain the hearing muſt be firſt reſtored: for as children learn to ſpeak only by imitating thoſe whom they hear, it cannot be expected

expected they should pronounce any word which they have never heard spoken.—Deafness from the womb is altogether incurable, and consequently the dumbness occasioned by it must be so too. The pretensions to teach those who are naturally deaf to speak, provided there is nothing wrong in the organs of speech, seems to be rather a piece of curiosity than any real utility. Our ingenious countryman, Dr. Wallis, was the inventor of this art, which was afterwards improved by Ammannus, a celebrated practitioner at Amsterdam: but with regard to its surprising success, we can say with the poet,

Write not what cannot be with ease conceiv'd ;
Some truths may be *too strong* to be *believ'd.*

When the fault in pronunciation proceeds from the ligament of the tongue being too short, or too thick, (or, as the popular phrase is, being *tongue-tied)* the remedy is very easy : but in the first place you must examine whether the ligament has this defect; and to convince yourself of that, you must try whether the child is able to thrust his tongue out of his mouth: if he cannot do so, you may be sure that the ligament is defective, and therefore it ought to be immediately cut: an operation that requires a person of skill ; for in cutting this ligament, care must be taken not to wound the two small veins running under the tongue, which is often of bad consequence, and sometimes chidren have been known to perish on the spot from an unskilful performance of the operation. A recent instance of which happened under the hands of a famous surgeon in Paris, in 1781, who, in cutting the ligaments of a child's tongue, inadvertently cut though one of these veins, which he did not take any notice of, but went away, as

L

soon as he saw the child begin to suck. After
sucking sufficiently, the nurse laid him in his
cradle, and he continued to move his lips, as if
he had been still sucking; but this was not particularly noticed, because many children have
such a motion when they are asleep. In the mean
time, what he sucked was the blood that came
out of the vein, and which he swallowed as fast
as it bled, the bleeding being still increased by
the motion of sucking. Thus he continued, till
there was no more blood left in his vessels, without
any thing amiss being perceived, 'till a little
before his death, when his paleness and weakness
indicated the cause.

The child was opened after his death, when
the stomach was found full of the blood which he
had swallowed.

We must not confound the *loss of the voice* with
dumbness; for as in the latter case the person cannot speak at all, in the former he can speak, but
only with a low voice. This loss of voice is often
owing to a viscid humour, which, sticking close
to the organs of the voice, and the neighbouring
parts, hinders the free vibrations and undulations
of the air, by which sound is produced. The cir-
cumstance of a wind instrument being besmeared
with any mucous liquor, whence it can only form
an obscure sound, is a representation of what
happens to us upon the loss of voice.

Many causes may contribute to this defect,
particularly severe colds, breathing an air too full
of dust, or impregnated with the smoke of candles,
lamps, &c. too acrid food, as salt-fish, cheese,
&c. straining the voice too much by public speaking, or singing, especially in the open air, or
being

being too suddenly expofed to the air afterwards, as is often the cafe on quitting convivial meetings at taverns, and entertainments of jollity.

The following remedies have been generally prefcribed for this defect.

1ft. A handful of great gourd-feeds blanched and dried; an equal quantity of cucumber feeds prepared in the fame manner; a dram of bole armoniac; two ounces of the root of mallows, frefh dug, and dried in an oven, with four ounces of brown fugar candy. Reduce them all to a powder, and take a little in your mouth every now and then.

2d. Frequently ufe lozenges of the following ingredients, letting them melt upon your tongue: —Take mucilage of gum tragacanth, prepared with rofe water, two ounces; bole armoniac, fix drams; root of the greater comfrey in powder, half an ounce; brown fugar-candy, a fufficient quantity, to make them into a due confiftence.

3d. Drink frequently of barley and liquorice water; eat black-currant jelly; and gargle the mouth twice or thrice every morning with the fyrup of mulberries, diluted with a glafs of milk-warm water; or with the fyrup of hedge-muftard, diluted the fame way.

4th. Bathe the feet frequently in warm water; and never expofe yourfelf, efpecially your head and breaft, to the cold.

There are women whofe voices refemble thofe of men; and there are men again, who fpeak with a woman's voice; as fome women have beards, and fome men have none. It is certainly very mortifying to a young lady to have a mafculine voice, and yet is a very frequent circumftance. It is

L 3   caufed

canfed by the extra-widenefs of the wind-
pipe ; in proportion to which, the voice will
be fmall and fhrill, or deep and hoarfe.——As
a means of contracting the larynx, you muft
drink nothing hot, but as cool as poffible. Frequently ufe lemonade, water acidulated with verjuice, oranges, &c. but in fmall mouthfuls at a
time, and flowly. Gargle the throat every morning with equal quantities of verjuice and water.—
Never fatigue yourfelf with much walking; and
fhun all difagreeable noifes, efpecially of fingers
who have a very horfe voice.

This is all that is practicable in regard of ladies
who have a mafculine voice. As to men whofe
voices refemble thofe of women, the following
rules may affift in giving them a more manly tone.

They fhould exercife their voice frequently in
finging bafe, which will contribute much to
ftrengthen it.—Conftantly in the mornings, at
rifing, pronounce the letters *A* and *O,* for fome
time, forming the found as deep in the throat as
poffible.——Apply the mouth to a hole in the
upper part of an empty hogfhead, and make it
echo to the voice, which muft be as hollow as
poffible.—Frequently read aloud.—Demofthenes
is faid to have ftrengthened his voice by declaiming
along the fea-fide, amid the noife of the billows.
Such methods muft be perfevered in for a length
of time, in order to have fuccefs.

Any other deficiencies of fpeech, or defects of
pronunciation, will be beft overcome by the example and affiftance of able teachers ; and the attentive perufal of the beft writers on elocution
and rhetoric.

HEBE.

H E B E.

B O O K III.

Of Correcting and Preventing Deformities in the Body.

FOLLOWING the divifion laid down in the firft book, we proceed to the trunk of the body; comprehending therein the fpine, cheft, loins, lower-belly, &c.

Of the Spine.

The fpine is that long chain of moveable bones placed one upon another, all along the back, from the top of the neck down to the rump, and compofing that flexible column upon which the head is placed, as upon an axis, with refpect to the firft vertebræ.

When the fpine is ftrait, well fet, and finely turned, it is a perfonal beauty; and when crooked or ill-formed, is no lefs a bodily deformity.

The upper part of the cheft is attached to the fpine above, and to the haunches below; fo that the fpine is a kind of trunk for compacting the whole body together; hence anatomifts compare

L 3   it

it to the keel of a ſhip, to which the ribs, the poop, the prow, and all the different parts of the veſſel are joined.

The ſpine begins below with a large baſis, and growing gradually more ſlender, it ends in a point at the top.

The upper part, which forms the neck, is nclined forward, and this gives the head a more ſtonvenient ſituation; for if the ſpine had been clraight in this place, the head would have reclined too far backwards.

· That part of the ſpine which makes the back, on the contrary, is turned outwards, whereby the capacity of the *thorax* is enlarged, and ſufficient ſpace is left for the lungs and heart, which is requiſite for their perpetual motion.

. That part of the ſpine which is towards the haunches is turned a little inwards, that it may counterbalance the weight of the body, and ſerve as a ſupporter to the parts above it; for if it had been turned outwards like the back, the body, which is principally ſupported by this part, could not have been kept ſtraight without great difficulty, but would have been almoſt quite inclined forwards.

That portion of the ſpine which is neareſt the rump, (and is formed of a large immovable bone, ſerving as a pedeſtal to the ſpine, and which anatomiſts call the *os ſacrum)* advances outwards, but more in women than in men.

The upper part of the cheſt, and the haunches, which are attached to the ſpine, are the eſſential parts of the body; ſo that if theſe parts are ill made, whether naturally or by accident, let the ſpine be never ſo ſtraight, the body in general cannot be perfect.

The

The cheſt is attached to the ſpine by the ribs. The external conformation of the cheſt, when it is well made and proportioned, is one of the greateſt beauties of the body. A high, full cheſt, has a pleaſing effect upon the eye, and adds much to perſonal dignity ; on the contrary, one that is flat and depreſſed is equally incompatible with health and beauty.

The cheſt on the upper part, immediately be- low the fore part of the neck, has two bones lying upon it, which are crooked outwards, and placed with their ends towards one another, one on each ſide, leaving a ſmall hollow in the place where they meet. The bending of theſe two bones (which are called the clavicles, and ſupport the arms) cauſes a conſiderable hollowneſs at the throat, much more remarkable in men than in women. It is obſervable that men move their arms with more eaſe than women, but this is compenſated for by the elegant form of the neck in the other ſex, is always the more graceful the leſs that theſe bones are arched. The clavicles are alſo longer in proportion as the arch is diminiſhed, whence wo- men commonly have the upper part of the breaſt larger, and conſequently the cheſt more beauti- ful : whence, too, we may obſerve, that women carry their arms much farther back than men.

As the beauty of the female boſom depends ſo much on the proper formation of theſe bones, we have been rather explicit in deſcribing them, and recommend a proper attention to parents, by no means to bind the ſhoulders of their chil- dren too tight, as this makes the clavicles grow crooked, and hence produces a contraction of the cheſt. For the ſame reaſon, as children grow up, their

their cloaths ought to be so made, as to allow them sufficient liberty to turn their arms outwards, besides encouraging them to thrust forward the chest, and accustoming them to the frequent use of such motion.

Under the clavicles lie the chest ; the fore part of which is a large flat bone called the sternum, performing the office of a breast-plate, and reaching from the fore-part of the neck to the pit of the stomach. To the two sides of the sternum, between the breasts, the ribs are attached, which bend backwards, towards the spine, and together with the sternum, make the cavity called the *thorax.*

The proportion of the haunches and belly contribute not a little to the beauty of shape, especially in women, who never have a fine waist, unless the haunches are a little raised. It is this elevation, or rather projection of the haunches, which produces that fine shape, that consists in a sensible decrease of the thickness of the body towards the haunches, especially on the sides ; or as Prior says,

———" that elegance of shape exprefs,
" Fine by degrees, and beautifully lefs."

A sort of beauty that seems almost destroyed by the present fashinable mode of dress.

To preserve the body straight requires strict attention from the earliest years. To prevent the bellies of children from advancing too much forwards, you must oblige them to sit upright. The same method must be used for keeping their

back

back ftraight; for if they fit with their body bent, the back will become crooked and round.

Another very neceffary precaution, is to take care that the bottom of the feat upon which they fit be not hollow in the middle, but quite plain. ——Hence timber chairs are to be preferred to thofe of ftraw or rufhes, which are unavoidably made with a hollow.

Shoes that are too high heeled, tight or fhort, are likewife very apt to diftort the bodies of children. Nor ought young ladies to be allowed either to few or read, but in an erect pofture, without which their bodies will infallibly become crooked : befides that nothing is more ungraceful than to fee young people ftooping to their books or needle.

The *piles* in children, from the pain they occafion, prevent them from keeping their body in an erect pofture, but caufe them to bend it different ways, till at laft a diftortion is brought on. A little of the herb *mercury,* and an equal quantity of *pellitory of the wall,* bruifed between the fingers, or in the hollow of the hand, and foftened with frefh butter, may be applied to the part affected ; and if continued for feveral days, does not repel the *hemorrhoids* (which, would be dangerous) but removes the pain, and difpofes to a difcharge, or elfe difcuffes them.

The bad confequences of tight, or mifhapen ftays, is too well known to need enlargement upon. We fhall only obferve, that when children are recovering from any diforder that has confined them to their beds, an attention to ftays becomes more particularly requifite; as the body then weakened by difeafe, will very readily affume any fhape. For when a perfon lies in bed, the bones

of the fpine do not prefs upon one another, neither
do they feel the weight of the head ; hence, after
fuch confinement in a recumbent pofture, the bones
recede from each other, and the body becomes
longer ; hence it requires fome time for the vertebræ to grow compact, and recover its ftrength
and firmnefs : while in the mean time diftortion
may be contracted.

The head ought, for gracefulnefs of body to be
carried ftraight, neither inclining to the one
fhoulder nor to the other, forwards nor backwards;
yet not in fuch an extreme as to make it and the
neck appear nailed to the fhoulders.—But to cut
fhort rules and directions on fuch a fubject, point
out elegant models to your children, praife thofe
models, and exhort them to imitation. There is
fo natural a defire in every perfon, even children, to
appear beautiful, that little exhortation will be
neceffary on this head ; and fhould *affectation* incline to an error on the other fide, it is perhaps
more eafily corrected, and certainly lefs difagreeable than the fault we fpeak of.

In general, to correct certain bodily deformities,
it may be proper to put in practice what a modern writer advifes for fubduing certain violent
paffions. " As thofe workmen, fays he, who make
ftraight wood crooked, are not content to bring
it to that point of ftraightnefs where they would
have it remain, but bend it farther to the other
fide, left the natural effort of the wood fhould recover its firft ftate ; fo one who would fubdue any
ftrong paffion, ought to incline to the other extreme, that he may be able to keep within thofe
bounds in which he defigns to confine himfelf."

No

No defpicable expedient for making children walk upright, when they come to five or fix years of age, is to encourage them to carry fomething light on their heads ; which may be eafily done when feveral of them are engaged in paftime, by raifing an emulation among them who fhall do it beft. The milk-maids in the country are never feen to ftoop, which can be attributed only to the burthens they carry on their heads.

Such expedients are greatly preferable to the ufe of fteel collars, or whale-bone machines ; which are fo irkfome to children, that when the reftraint is removed, they frequently practice the diftortion through contradiction.

In fome children, the neck is fo crooked, or ftiff, that it is impoffible for them to move it when they would : a defect fometimes occafioned by accidents in the delivery ; and which the phyfician or midwife will properly know how to correct.

When the deformity comes afterwards, it is frequently owing to an ill cuftom of allowing the child to hold his head too long, and too often, to one fide of the cradle, attracted perhaps by the light, or fome glittering object ; in order to gaze at which he violently ftrains the mufcles of his head and neck, till thofe parts take a fet that way. The rheumatifm, too, may occafion it ; which a cold wind, received upon any part of the neck, is capable of producing.

When the complaint proceeds from ill habit, the removal of the caufe will accelerate the cure, which may be affifted by taking the child's head gently between your hands, turning it by degrees

to

to the oppofite fide, and this ought to be repeated every now and then.

If the deformity proceeds from a rheumatifm in the neck, it may be frequently well rubbed with oil of nutmegs, and kept very warm.

An attention to the operations of nature may be of fervice in this cafe : obferve how fhe acts in plants. You fee a little fhrub fet in a window, with all its branches turned to one fide—obferve how foon it tuins them to the other, after you change its fituation. The whole fhrub twifts about, and is obedient to the air, which attracts it to the other fide. This change is the invifible effort of nature operating within the plant. Something fimilar happens in the human body.

I recollect a very appofite circumftance which happened at the laft difplay of fireworks on Tower hill. A girl of ten years old, who had had her neck crooked from the age of feven, the deformity having come on by degrees, was unexpectedly cured of it, after this manner :—Her mother took her to a houfe to fee the diverfion, where the windows were fituated in fuch a manner, that it could only be feen on one fide ; and this being the fide oppofite whereto the child's head was turned, curiofity caufed her to make fuch violent efforts to turn herfelf to the other, where the exhibition was, that it feemed to her as if one had been pulling her head from her fhoulders : the ftrong defire, however, of viewing the fpectacle, made her neglect the pain ; and every time fhe heard the explofion of the gun-powder, or the acclamations of the populace, fhe redoubled her efforts. In fhort, fhe ftruggled fo much, that before the rejoicing was over, fhe could

turn

turn her head either to the right or left with very little pain, which in a few days entirely vanifhed.

This may be a hint to parents who have children in a fimilar predicament. For though fire-works are not always at hand to accomplifh this effect, yet many other plans may be invented. When the child is feated at table, place yourfelf on that fide moft difficult for him to turn to ; fpeak to him frequently in fuch a way as he fhall be obliged to anfwer you, and make an effort to look at you. Lay upon your chair fomething that he likes, and afk him if he will have it. Such proceeding will make him endeavour to turn his neck towards you : and repeated efforts will moft probably be crowned with fuccefs.

It will be proper, while purfuing thefe means, frequently to rub that fide of the neck to which the head inclines, with emollients and fpirituous liquors : or take equal parts of the oil of worms and brandy, mix, and let them be applied warm.

The neck, to be well fhaped, muft be round and moderately long and flender ; but at the fame time it ought to have a fort of plumpnefs or fullnefs, fo that the *pomum adami* may not ap-pear, efpecially in women.

There cannot be a more difagreeable blemifh (and it is genera ly a confpicuous one) on this part, than the *King's Evil*, or the *Bronchocc'e*. The former is as well known as its cure is difficult. Too much attention cannot be paid to the nurfe's milk : as little dependance can be had upon me-dicinal application at fo early a period. Nothing, perhaps, can be fafer than a courfe of Ethiop's mi-neral and rhubarb, in the infant ftage of life.

M   In

In more advanced life, you may have recourfe to the following compound.

Take quickfilver, half a pound ; crude antimony, fix ounces ; fulphur, two ounces ; rub thefe two or three hours in an iron mortar, till they are reduced into an impalpable powder, and tie them in a rag: then take guiaicum, four ounces; faffafras, half a pound ; yellow fanders, caffamunair, zedoary and cinnamon, each an ounce ; juniper berries, fix ounces ; coriander feeds, two ounces ; leaves of agrimony, ground pine, St. John's wort, horfe-hound, fage, and buckbean, each two handfuls ; millipedes, half a pound ; let the woods, with the Ethiop's, boil in eight gallons of wort, till reduced to fix ; and while that is in fermentation, let the other ingredients hang in it.

All that a medicine in this form can promife in the moft obftinate cafes, this will perform, if duly continued ; the whole concurring with a united force to penetrate into, deterge and fcour every veffel, gland or cel: of the whole body. There are no diforders of the glands, how remote foever, that this will not wear away ; and even where the body is almoft one continued fore, this may be depended upon, if carefully followed. In fhort the whole circle of practice cannot produce a more efficacious, and a more convenient prefcription; there being not one fuperfluous article, or that diftaftes, or renders the medicine naufeous. —Drink half a pint every day.

Thofe to whom malt liquor is not agreeable, may contrive the above with wine, by letting the ingredients ftand longer in it, viz for fome weeks, and fometimes fhaking the veffel, but giving it a little vent at fuch times for fear of burfting.—It
may

may also be managed into a *hydromel* or *mead*; and for such to whom honey is not disagreeable, it may be the better, because it will be more defensive.

The *bronchocele* is a tumour rising in the fore part of the neck, from some humour, or other violence, as straining in labour, lifting of weights, &c. It is frequently called a *Derby-neck*, from the inhabitants of that county being much subject to it; probably for the same reasons that the inhabitants about the valleys of the Alps and other mountainous countries are so much affected with it, namely the air and waters of the country. But it has not yet been explained in what manner they operate to produce these effects.

This tumour, when once become inveterate, is very difficultly, if at all, curable by medicines; but may be dispersed if it is recent. A leaden collar, mixed with mercury, prevents it from growing bigger, if it does not entirely disperse it. The most celebrated remedy is one sold at Coventry, but kept a secret by the preparer. It is ordered to be laid under the tongue every night at going to bed.

A fair bosom is too principal an object among the ladies to pass here unnoticed: we have described the essentials of it in the former part of this work, and now will endeavour to give some assistance in correcting its defects.

To make the neck and bosom very fair, the following wash is much celebrated.

Take fumitory water, and dew gathered in May, or the beginning of June, each a quarter of a pint; oil or spirit of lavender, two ounces; chymical oil of mace, one dram; Benjamin water,

four

four ounces: mix them together ; and having firſt
waſhed the neck and boſom with a compoſition
of equal parts of chamomile water and white wine
as warm as may be, dip a fine cloth in the other,
with which waſh yourſelf a ſecond time The
uſe of this for a few weeks will make a conſiderable change in the complexion.

A modern writer, * in deſcribing the manners
of the Aſiatic ladies, obſerves, that " nothing can
exceed the care they take to preſerve their breaſts
as the moſt ſtriking mark of beauty. In order
to prevent them from growing large or ill-
ſhaped, they incloſe them in caſes made of exceedingly *light wood*, which are joined together and
faſtened with buckles of jewels behind. Theſe
caſes are ſo ſmooth and pliant, that they yield to
the attitudes of the body without being flattened,
or without the ſmalleſt injury to the delicacy of
the ſkin." The writer has not been pleaſed to
name the *ſort* of *wood* the Aſiatics employ ; but
the Engliſh ladies may not be diſpleaſed to learn
the following method of bringing to a firm plump-
neſs and roundneſs ſuch breaſts as hang down or
appear too large.

Bind them up cloſe with linen caps or bags that
will juſt fit them, and let them continue ſo for ſix
or eight days.

Take carrot-ſeed, aniſe, fennel, and plantane,
ſeeds, each two ounces ; virgin honey, an cunce
and a half; the juice of plantane, and vinegar, each
two ounces ; bruiſe the ſeeds groſsly, and put
them into the liquid, ſtirring them well together:
at the expiration of the above time, take off the
caps and anoint the breaſts with the oil of ſavin ;

after

* Travels in Aſia and Africa, publiſhed in 1782.

after which fpread the compofition on a linen
cloth, and lay it on, fo that it may cover the
breafts, putting the fame caps over them again,
and binding them up as ftraight as confiftent
with your eafe : on the fourth day, take all
off, and wafh your breafts with warm whi e wine
and rofe water, continuing fo to do morning and
evening for twelve or fourteen days; when you
will find them reduced to an elegant roundnefs,
firm and plump.

There are feveral other perfonal deformities
which feem principally owing to negleft in the
attention of parents and nurfes, though they
may fometimes be natural defecls ; viz.
　1ft. The neck funk between the fhoulders,
　2d. One fhoulder higher or thicker than the
other.
　3d. The fhoulder inclining too much to the
one fide :
　Of thefe we fhall take a curfory review.

To hinder the fhoulders from growing round,
care muft be taken to keep the elbows well back,
placed over the haunches, and the cheft forward.
The perfon fhould lie as flat in bed as poffible,
and if one fhoulder is too thick, he ought always
to fleep on the oppofite fide : for th fhoulder upon which one refts, always projects beyond the
plane of the back.

Writing upon tables either too high or too low,
expofes to the fame fault, or to that of being round
fhouldered. When you obferve that a child inclines to fink his neck between his fhoulders, you
fhould never allow him to fit upon an elbow chair,
for while refting his arms upon the elbows, his fhoulders rife, and of courfe his neck finks between them.

When the fhoulder inclines too much to one
fide, the *left* for example, let the child often ftand
upon the *right* foot alone ; for in fupporting him-

felf upon this foot, while the other remains inactive, it neceffarily happens that the right fhoulder, which was too high, muft fall lower; and the left fhoulder, which was too low, muft be raifed higher This is evident from the neceffity of fupporting the body in an equilibrium.

Another method is, to carry a little burthen upon the fhoulder that is loweft, and let the higheft quite alone; for the weight upon the low fhoulder will oblige him to raife it up, and at the fame time will make him deprefs the other.—Contrary to the opinion and practice of thofe, who lay a weight upon the higheft fhoulder, imagining the weight will make him deprefs it, while in fact it only makes him raife it higher.

A very eafy method is, to bend your arm, and fet your hand on your fide; the fhoulder of that fide will be raifed, and the other will fink lower, efpecially if you let the hand of the other fall as low down by the thigh as you can. This is a very fimple expedient, and may be practiced without any one gueffing the defign.

Many people have a habit, when they write, or kneel down to prayers, of drawing in the cheft, pulling down the fhoulders, and folding the arms over the ftomach; this infenfibly brings on a deformity, which gives the body, in its upper and pofterior parts, a figure like the back of a fpoon.

To correct this deformity, the practice muft be laid afide, and fuch a pofture affumed as is oppofite to that by which it is contracted; advancing the cheft; throwing back the fhoulders, and letting the hands fall down by the fides.—Attention only is required. Probably, learning the military exercife might prove as certain a corrective as any that could be prefcibed.

The

The back *hunched*, *hollow*, or *crooked*, are the effects of an ill-shaped fpine, which may proceed either from a fall, or an effort to lift too heavy burthens, as often happens to children in attempting to carry each other. This diſtortion of the fpine is either outward or inward, or both together. When outward, it makes the hunch back ; when inwards, the hollow back ; and when both ways, it makes the crooked back, refembling the fhape of the letter *S*. The hunch is frequently on the fore part of he cheft, forming a fharp point, fomething like that rifing which is to be obferved upon the breaft of an old fowl, to which it is commonly compared.

If early attended to, the hunch, as well of the *ſternum* as the back, may be corrected, by frequent gentle preffures of the hand ; obferving at the fame time to rub the parts with the oil of nutmeg. The ufe of whale-bone bodice, gently to comprefs the part that hunches out, is of great fervice here. In the mean time, let the child's bed be not too foft, without any bolfter, and make him lie frequently upon his back, fo that the head and fpine may be as much upon a direct line with one another as poffible.

The crookednefs of the fpine does not always proceed from a fault in itfelf, but may be occafioned by the mufcles of the fore part of the body being too fhort : in which cafe external medicines, fuch as the oil of worms, decoction of mallows, marfh mallows &c. muft be applied from the top of the cheft to the bottom of the belly. The latter caufe may be difcover d by a particular ſtiffnefs and tenſion in the parts. When the mufcles are foftened by the above applications,

they

they will relax, and allow the fpine to recover its due fhape.

When the fpine is crooked inwards, you muft make the child ftoop frequently, by throwing cards, pictures, &c. upon the floor ; and the pofture into which he will be obliged to put himfelf, will at length force the hollow part outwards.

When the fpine is crooked in the form of an *S*, it is beft to have recourfe to whalebone bodice, ftuffed in fuch a manner that the ftuffed parts fhall exactly anfwer to thofe protuberances which you wifh to reprefs; and thefe bodice muft be renewed every three months at leaft.

It is very neceffary to obferve, that in proportion as the protuberances diminifh, the ftuffing muft be increafed.—A circumftance that requires fuch very ftrict and nice attention as few but parents are capable of.

The deformity of which we have been fpeaking, is frequently occafioned by the *rickets*; on the treatment of which we do not mean to enter, farther than to fuggeft a new, and perhaps very advantageous method of procedure.

Without-having recourfe to the various machines propofed for exercifing rickety children, you can do nothing better than every morning to fprinkle their face with cold water, in the fame manner as when you would recover a perfon from a fainting fit. The fright from this fudden application obliges them to exert fuch motions as contribute furprifingly to reftore the former fhape of the deformed parts. The fame effect will be experienced from applying a linen cloth, dipt in white wine to the arms, from the wrift to the el-

bow

rubbing them afterwards with a very dry towel. This puts all the mufcles of the body into motion, and the *vifcera* themfelves will partake of the fhock. One can fcarcely believe how efficacious thefe motions are : and how much fuperior their effect is, to all the exercife that can be procured by fwings, and fimilar machines.

The fuccefs will be greater by rubbing the fpine, from the nape of the neck to the hip, and all along the thighs down to the heels, with a linen cloth, dipped either in white wine, or weak brandy and water ; always taking care to wipe them with a dry linen cloth.

Tickling the foles of the feet in rickety children is looked upon as a good expedient; for it throws them into motions which they would not otherwife make ufe of, and which are fometimes fo effectual as to make the body recover its natural fhape.

When the bodies of children or adults become deformed from a luxation or fracture, the cure is very difficult, and requires the affiftance of the ableft medical practitioners. When the deforty is caufed by an obftruction, the fpine fhould be chafed with volatile and fp'rituous fomentations, to diffipate the obftruction.

Corpulency, when it is no greater than to come under the French denomination *d' être embon point*, is fo far from a deformity, as to be rather confidered as a perfection: an unwieldy groffnefs is, however, very difgufting, efpecially when it appears to proceed from the practice of *kitchen* philofophy. The beft way to remedy this over-bulkinefs, is to be very temperate in eating and drinking, efpecially wine, beer, chocolate, and fuch

ſuch nutritive diet; not to indulge many hours
in ſleep; drink freely of tea and coffee; take a good
deal of exerciſe on foot; and laſtly, take every
day, for ſome weeks, a dram of the aſhes of cray-
fiſh, mixed with a freſh egg, or diluted with
breth. But if the diſpoſition to grow corpulent
is ſo very predominant as to require more powerful attenuants, to any quantity of the above aſhes
you may add equal parts of thoſe of *ſea ſpunge*, and
of the pith of ſweet briar; make them into a powder, of which half a dram is a doſe.

This preparation is ſo very attenuating, that
it may ſometimes cauſe too great meagerneſs, unleſs particular regard is had to the diſpoſition of
the perſon who takes it: for unleſs he is afraid of
growing to an enormous ſize, the former medicine
ought to be preferred.

Many young people, to abate their bulkineſs,
and procure themſelves an eaſy ſhape, uſe vinegar
with every thing they eat, and ſometimes even
drink it. The remedy is highly dangerous, and
the leaſt miſchief it can do, is to render them
conſumptive.

A young lady, who enjoyed a very perfect ſtate
of health till the age of eighteen, with a good
appetite and a blooming complexion, began to be
ſuſpicious of growing too fat, eſpecially as her
mother was corpulent: a woman, with whom ſhe
conſulted on this ſubject, adviſed her to drink
every day a ſmall glaſs of vinegar: ſhe did ſo accordingly, and her bulkineſs diminiſhed. Pleaſed
with the ſucceſs of her remedy, ſhe continued it
more than a month: at length ſhe began to have
a cough; and as it was dry at firſt, it was looked
upon only as a ſlight cold, which would go off
again. In the mean time, from a dry cough, it
came

came to a spitting, a fever succeeded, with difficulty of breathing, and her whole habit of body became lean and consumptive. Night sweats came on, with swellings of the legs and feet, and the disease ended with a diarrhoea, of which she expired.

On dissection, the lobes of the lungs were found full of tubercles :—the lungs resembled a grape, and the tubercles the stones.—During her illness, the Peruvian bark was administered, as also febrifuge and alkaline opiates, the whey of asses milk, and broth of cray-fish ; to which were added the pectoral herbs, to prevent an ulceration of the lungs.—But in spite of medicine, the consumption continued its course.*

Too great slenderness is a deformity which we have less cause to be alarmed at, than the opposite extreme. Children, at a certain time, necessarily become lean, viz. when they begin to increase sensibly in their stature. This leanness need therefore give a parent no concern, as it is only temporary.—But when children fall into it from fretting, or some secret chagrin, they insensibly pine away till the nutritive substance is quite exhausted, and the body becomes like a skeleton ;—the face will sometimes preserve an appearance of plumpness, while the other parts of the body, particularly the back-bone and ribs, become emaciated.

It will often be found that this leanness, or rather decline of health, is owing to a latent grief, or to jealousy, at seeing either a child, or some other object, more noticed and indulged than itself. One can scarcely imagine how painfully sensible children are of this partiality ; they possess
an

*Edinburgh Medical Essays.

an extraordinary inftinct, or fenfibility, (call it by what name you pleafe) and are powerfully agitated by all thofe paffions which tend to the prefervation of *felf*. They conceal their grief, and it fometimes requires fkill and management to difcover the caufe.

The readieft way is to fhew lefs fondnefs for the fuppofed object of jealoufy; and if this be the occafion of his anxiety, you will foon perceive the child lefs fullen and melancholy, and his eyes begin again to fparkle with pleafure. As foon as the fecret is difcovered, you muft refolve, to re-trench all the careffes which you ufed to give others before him, and fhew the greateft fondnefs poffible for him, but in fuch a manner that he may not difcover the trick ; for children are often artful enough to pry into the very breafts of thofe that are about them ; and indeed, in this fenfe we often become their dupes. From this renewed fondnefs, his heart will be foon reftored to peace, and he will daily recover health, ftrength, and fpirits.

The body feems fometimes all of a thicknefs, without any thing free or eafy about it; and though it is otherwife well enough fhaped, yet has fuch a conftrained air, as if the perfon had a ftake thruft up his body. This might be prevented or corrected by a freedom of exercife, particularly in fuch diverfions as oblige a perfon to jump much; as that action makes the body form a variety of angles that are of great fervice towards giving it an air of freedom.

Indeed in every cafe where exercife can be ufed, it will be found of the higheft advantage in affift-ing the cure of bodily deformities; or rendering the misfortune lefs oppreffive, by contributing to the general welfare of the fyftem. In preventing
and

and curing a number of difeafes, there is nothing
equal to moderate exercife: It roufes the natural
heat, diffipates fuperfluours humours, gives agility
to the mufcles, ftrengthens the nerves, opens the
pores, and affifts perfpiration. Hence the whole
body muft be invigorated, the fenfes rendered
quicker, refpiration more free, and the breaft and
ftomach more ftrong and vigorous.

Do you wifh that a woman fhould have a happy delivery?—nothing is better for this purpofe
than moderate exercife in the fifth, fixth, and
feventh months of pregnancy. Would you difpofe
children to fleep, and eafe thofe pains with which
they are fo often troubled?---nothing is more
effectual for this, than rocking them in the cradle.
—Would you prevent or cure the rickets?—you
can ufe no better remedy than conftantly toffing
them in your arms, rolling him about, and throwing
their limbs and body into a variety of motions.—
Would you ftrengthen the tone of the ftomach,
and in fhort of the whole body? This is to be
done by riding, and dancing, which laft exercife
both ftrengthens the legs and feet, and renders
their joints more flexible: It is no lefs agreeable
than conducive to health; makes the body active,
the mind chearful, the complexion lively, and
gives the face and whole body a graceful mien
and air. If you wifh to render the body ftrong
and fit to endure hardfhips, ftrengthen the vital
actions, and reduce the habit when it is too corpulent;—have recourfe to the more active diverfions of tennis, cricket, fives, fkittles; or the
more laborious ones of rowing, digging, ringing
bells, and fuch athletic fports. For it is to thefe
employments, that the labouring clafs of people in
general owe their exemption from many difeafes

N   that

that are the conftant attendants upon the luxury and indolence of higher life.

Walking puts the whole body into motion, and hence is not only of fervice to the lower extremities, but clears the lungs, ftrengthens the ftomach, and is of great relief to gravelly complaints: and is certainly the beft exercife for the very young and the aged; as fencing, hunting, courfing, &c. are more adapted to the prime of life. Singing, reading, and talking aloud, may be reckoned among the beft kind of exercifes; for by the exertion of the voice, the animal fpirits are all put into motion, from the very fountain from whence they arife; and it may perhaps be owing to the natural difpofition to the two former, that women do not ftand fo much in need of other active exercife as men. Exercife, in a word, is fo ufeful and neceffary, that not only man, but the moft inactive and indolent of the brute creation,—nay even plants and vegetables cannot thrive without it. The humble violet, as well as the lofty oak, loves to be agitated by the winds. And we ough to admire the clemency of Divine juftice, which, in chaftifing man for his fins, has condemned him to fuch a punifhment as conduces the moft to preferve his health.

BOOK III. PART II.

Of the Deformities of the Arms, Hands, Legs, and Feet.

WHEN a perfon is born with one arm, or leg fhorter or longer than the other, or with knots, crook dn is, or diftortions upon them, the cafe is incurable; when the deformity is occafioned by violence in the delivery, or by aukwardnefs in the *accoucheur*, fome relief may be expected.

When in a new-born infant, the *pelvis* feems awry, you have very juft caufe to fufpect that this deformity in refpect of the length of the leg, is occafioned by fome pull which the child has fuffered by the hand of the midwife; and a cure may be effected by replacing the pelvis in its natural fituation. But if the leg appears too long, while the pelvis is not awry, you may be fure that there is a natural fault in the conformation of the leg, in which cafe the deformity is not to be helped.

What is here faid of the leg when it is too long, may be alfo underftood of it when too fhort; for if one fide of the pelvis be pufhed up by any violence, the thigh and leg of that fide muft be thruft up higher, and appear fhorter.

The fame doctrine holds true of the arms; for tho' they cannot be in readily made longer, yet in

pulling

pulling the arm, the midwife may make the spine incline too much to one side, whereby the arm of that side will reach farther down, though not really longer than it was before.

To reduce the pelvis, when the leg appears too long,—stretch the child out upon his back, and tie a small handkerchief, doubled into several folds, loosely about the knee of the leg which appears too long, in manner of a garter; to this handkerchief, at the external part of the knee, tie a pretty large fillet, about two ells in length, and fasten it as tight as he can bear (but without hurting him) about the child's shoulder, of the same side; taking care that it be tied in such manner as not to slip, and then swathe him up. The compression which the swaddling-band makes upon the other, which is stretched from the knee to the shoulder, will make the latter more tense; and by increasing the tension, determine that side of the pelvis, which was too low to rise up; and the situation of the pelvis, from being oblique, will become horizontal, and consequently recover its natural position.

If the deformity has been neglected till the child is grown up, you may put him into a pair of tight bodice, which will have the same effect with the swaddling-band upon the bandage that reaches from the knee to the shoulder.

The thigh or leg may be luxated from the womb, by different causes, as may also other parts of the body, as the shoulder, elbow, heels, &c. in all which cases, immediate recourse must be had to the hand of a surgeon; for, if neglected, a callus will be formed in the dislocated part, which will render the cure absolutely impossible.

" A

" A young lady, who had diſlocated her thigh, and neglected calling in proper aſſiſtance, was an inſtance of the misfortune juſt mentioned: a callus formed by degrees, and rendered uſeleſs all the aſſiſtance which could be got afterwards, and ſhe remained crooked. But a circumſtance ſomewhat ſingular happened on this occaſion, that ſhe bore three boys with each of them a thigh luxated, and who continued cripples; while three girls, to whom ſhe was alſo mother, were ſtrong and wellmade." *Zuing. Theatr. Pr. Med.*

When an arm or a leg are ſhort by contraction of the muſcles, or being withered, let the part be firſt well rubbed with a piece of coarſe cloth, or a fleſh-bruſh, but not too roughly ; then anointed with juniper-butter, and wrapt up in a linen cloth Theſe frictions and unguent muſt be continued ſeveral weeks, or even months.

The juniper butter is thus prepared :

Melt a pound of freſh butter, and mix with it a ſmall handful of large, black, freſh juniper berries, bruiſed only between the fingers, and not ſo as to break the hard ſtones within them, which would make the butter acrid : then boil it upon a gentle fire, and when theſe ſtones are become ſoft, put the mixture into a linen cloth, and ſqueeze it ſtrongly, to preſs out the ointment into a glaſs veſſel.

The application of *currier*'s oil to relax the muſcles, and wearing a ſhoe with a leaden ſole, (the weight of which is proportioned to the contraction) is preſcribed for the ſame deformity, but muſt be continued for a long time.

An

An arm, a leg, a hand, or a foot, is sometimes
slenderer than the other, for want of receiving
sufficient nourishment, while the other preserves
its natural state. This deformity may be corrected by the same means with the former, namely, y friction, and the juniper butter by way of
liniment

It sometimes happens, that not only one leg, or
one arm, but both arms, or both legs, receive less
nourishment than is necessary, and become shape-
less, or like spindles, while the rest of the body
appears in good condition. So far as external remedies can avail, those above described are the
properest, joined to a moderate share of walking.

The tendon which reaches from the calf of the
leg to the heel, is sometimes so short, that the
person is obliged to walk upon the fore-part of his
foot, without being able to set the heel to the
ground ; which not only obliges him to walk un-
gracefully, but is likewise fatiguing.

This defect is sometimes tolerably well palliated by high-heeled shoes, when both feet are in
this predicament ; but when one heel only is affected, the deformity is more obvious, from the
inequality of the shoe-heels. If the tendons are
not maimed, a cure may be obtained by relaxing
the parts with rubbing the leg from the ham to
below the heel, evening and morning, with the
oil of worms, after first exciting a kindly warmth
and motion by friction or the flesh-brush. The
leg may be frequently bathed in a bucket of tripe-
broth, moderately warm. To render such assistance yet more effectual, the person should exercise
himself frequently with climbing some pretty steep
hills.

hills. He may likewife have his fhoe-heel made of lead.

We have mentioned already, that the arms, to be handfome, ought to be round, fl fh , and a little flat in the infide, incealing gr d ally in thicknefs from the wrift almoft to the jo nt of the elbow.

The hand fhould be delicate, pretty long, and not fquare; the back of it ought to be a little plump, fo that the veins may not be very confpicuous, nor appear ftarting; and at the root of the finger there ought to be a fmall dimple when the hand is opened. The fingers long, not deftitute of flefh, a lit le round above, and flat below, with a certain air of freedom and motion, which ought to be confpicuous even when they are at reft.

When the hands are well fhaped, and delicate in fize and complexion, they are one of the greateft ornaments to female beauty.—Mary, Queen of Scots, whofe charms are a darling th me with hiftorians, was particularly remarked for the uncommon elegance and matchlefs fplendor of her hands and arms. Though fuch an ornament muft be purely the work of nature, yet it requires fome degree of care to preferve it; and with fimilar care we may alfo preferve the hands free from certain deformities, when they are not expofed to the feverity of labour.

The roughnefs of the hand confifts in the hardnefs of the fkin, which in labouring people is neither a matter of furprize, nor even a deformity, though it is certainly fuch in thofe whofe rank or profeffion exempts them from drudgery. Too much expofure to the air, dabbling frequently in very warm, or very cold water, or often wafhing

them

them with the common kinds of foap, have all the
fame effect in breaking the texture of the fkin, and
giving a look of coarfenefs and rufticity to the
hand. Too often and too long wafhing the
hands, makes them become chopped, and takes
away that livelinefs of the fkin, which is its peculiar beauty, but which is rather increafed than
deftroyed by fimply rubbing the hand either with
a foft cloth, or one againft the other; that delicate
moifture being fupplied by the finer cutaneous vef-
els, is too quickly exhaled by very warm water,
while the veff. ls are fhut up, and the exhalation re-
pelled by the ufe of very cold.

The fame preventives muft be confidered alfo
as correctives; to which may be added, rubbing
the hands every night with a little oil of eggs,
and putting on a pair of gloves; wafhing them
in the morning with a piece of ftale bread foaked
in wine and water; powder of bitter almonds,
oatmeal, flower of peafe, beans, &c. or the following ointment, may ferve for the above purpofe:

Take equal quantities of cream and bears-
greafe; virgin wax, a fufficient or proportionable
quantity; incorporate them all together over a
flow fire, and rub your hands with this ointment
every night, wearing gloves, and wafhing them
with a little water and white wine luke-warm.

Wafh-Balls.

Take of the beft white foap half a pound, and
fhave it into thin flices; then take two ounces and
a half of Florentine orrice root, three quarters
of an ounce of calamus aromaticus, and the fame
quantity of elder flowers; of cloves, one dram;
dried rofe leaves, half an ounce; coriander feeds,
lavender,

lavender, and bay leaves, each a dram ; with three
drams of ftorax ; reduce the whole to a fine powder, which knead into a pafte with the foap, adding a few grains of mufk or ambergreafe. It
may be ufed as a pafte ; or made into wafh-balls,
by foftening it with a little oil of almonds, to render the compofition more lenient. Too much
cannot be faid in favour of this wafh-ball, in regard of its cleanfing and cofmetic quality.

There are fome people whofe hands not only,
but whofe fkin in general, is fo exceeding coarfe
and rough, as to refemble that of the fea-dog ; a
deformity that proceeds from a fharp humour
fupplied by the cutaneous veffels, which fpreads
itfelf over all the furface of the hand, frets the
texture of the fkin, and raifes it up into little
fcales, refembling a file or a grater.

Others have their hands chopped, or full of
little chinks, frequently filled with matter, and
creating a very difagreeable blemifh.—This is
fometimes occafioned by the feverity of the weather during winter, and as often proceeds from
neglecting to dry the hands after wafhing.

The means of preventing thefe two laft deformities, is carefully to fhun what we have remarked
to be the caufe of them. To correct them, you
may have recourfe to fome of the following preparations.

The oil of wheat, extracted by an iron prefs, in
the fame manner as oil of almonds, is excellent for
chops in the hands, and rigidity of the fkin.

Or, beat fome peeled apples (having firft taken
out the cores) in a marble mortar, with equal
quantities of rofe-water and white wine :—add
fome bread-crumb, blanched almonds, and a little
white

white foap:—fimmer the whole over a flow fire till it acquires a proper confiftence.

Or, dry before the fire half a pound of bitter almonds blanched, then beat them in a marble mortar as fine as poffible, adding a little boiled milk to prevent the almonds from turning oily. In the fame manner beat the crumb of two French bricks, with four yolks of eggs boiled hard; and with the addition of fome frefh milk, kneed them into a pafte, which incorporate with that of the almonds.

Or, take of the flour of beans and lupins, well ground and finely fifted, each four ounces; white ftarch, orris, and blanched almonds, each two ounces; beat them together into a pafte, with four ounces of Caftile foap, and rofe water. This is excellent for making the hands foft and fmooth.

Among a great many deformities, or which go under' this name, there is a contraction, or feeble and indolent folding in of the fingers of the hand, with a lofs of the voluntary motion of thofe fingers, which remain folded in a negligent manner, and cannot be extended without the affiftance of the other hand, or of fome other perfon, and return to their former crookednefs fo foon as left to themfelves. This weaknefs proceeds from a relaxation of the mufcles of the hands; and, as phyficians tell us, is frequently the effects of a bilious and convulfive cholic which has preceded it.

The hand may alfo be crooked by fome external accident, as when the nerves or tendons are cut by a wound, withered and deftroyed by burning, or eroded by an ulcer; in which cafe the deformity is incurable.—But in the former cafe, when owing to a relaxation of the mufcles, great benefit may be derived from fuch external remedies as the following

lowing. Soaking the hand in the blood of an ox, calf, or fheep, as foon as killed, and repeating the operation as often as convenient; rubbing the hand and arm alfo with foft linen cloths a little warm, and afterwards with the oil of worms made moderately hot. When this courfe has been practifed for a fortnight, or longer, you may proceed to pump the parts with wine in this manner: namely, having a large earthen veffel with a hole near the bottom to admit a brafs cock, fill it with white wine made pretty warm, with the addition of a little cinnamon: fet this ciftern upon a high table, and let the perfon place his hand and arm fo as to receive the ftream of the wine, having another veffel underneath to receive it, as it muft be referved for further ufe.

This pumping fhould be continued for half an hour at a time, and repeated twice a-day.

If wine fhould be thought too expenfive, a preparation of the fame intention, and to be ufed as the foregoing, may be made with oak-bark, one pound; balauftines and red rofes dried, each fix handfuls; boil them in four gallons of water to two; ftrain, and add a quart of rough red wine; to which may be added alfo three ounces of alum. It muft be applied as hot as conveniently can be born.

Purgatives are indifpenfibly requifite to be joined with thefe external medicines.

The veins upon the back of the hand ought not to be too large and confpicuous, as when fo, the hand, however well fhaped, cannot be called beautiful: and where the hands are not employed in rough work, that propels the blood too plentifully to the veffels thereof, the blemifh may be eafily

prevented

prevented and even conected. Every thing muft be
avoided that can force the blood in too great quantities to the hands, or ftop it when there, as wafhing
in water too warm; keeping them too long hanging
down; wearing waiftcoats, ftays, or bodice too
tight below the arm-pits; for thefe prefs upon the
veffels under the arms, and, hindering the blood
from returning, make the veins of the hands to
fwell. You muft likewife wear nothing tight
about the wrifts or elbows; this producing the
fame effect as tying the arm with a ligature when
we want to be let blood : You fhould accuftom
yourfelf always to wear gloves, as they prefs gently
upon the veins, and prevent their being too much
filled with blood.

In the defect we have be n fpeaking of, as well
as in fome other blemifhes, as when the hand is
fwelled, red, or of any difagreeable colour, the
following compofition may be fuccefsfully ufed.

In a quart of white wine boil rofemary and
lavender-flowers each an ounce; penny royal and
rue, each a handful, dill and coriander feeds grofsly
bruifed, each a quarter of an ounce; ftrain out
the liquid, with which, moderately warm, wafh
your hands and arms.

Take barley meal, two ounces; juice of citrons,
one ounce; cream of tartar, oil of turpentine,
litharge of filver, and oil of rofes, each two drams;
make thefe ingredients into a falve over a gentle
fire, and apply it as a plaifter to the fingers and
hands, renewing it every other day for eight or
ten days.

This will reprefs any knots, or gouty appear-
ances on the hands or fingers, and reftore them to
an elegant neatnefs of fhape.

Such,

Such trifling tumours, as *warts* and *corns*, (efpecially the latter,) are often attended with much
pain; and it fometimes even requires the fkill of
a phyfician to ged rid of thofe troublefome ap-
pendages.

Every one knows thefe excrefcences fo well,
that they need little or no defcription; only that
warts are fmooth, or jagged, almoft flat with the
fkin, or more prominent, even to hanging down.

If they are not rooted in the tendons, but lie
in the fkin, they may eafily be cured, or taken
away. But if they rife from the former,
they can fcarcely be rooted out without danger.

There are various ways of deftroying warts, as
tying, cutting, or confuming them. Tying is
only for thofe of a certain fize, and which have
a very fmall ftalk: It is done by a ligature of filk,
or horfe hair. They may alfo be cut off: but
this ought cautioufly to be attempted; and they
very often grow again much larger than before.
They may be confumed by fome corrofive liquor,
as fpirit of falt, aqua fortis, fpirit of hartfhorn,
&c. and the laft will certainly be found the fafeft:
but in trying this method, you fhould apply a
plaifter to the hand, with holes to let the warts
pafs through, and prevent the application from
hurting the fkin.

A numerous tribe of medicines are offered for
removing thefe excrefcencies, and perhaps not
one of them can be recommended with much af-
furance of fuccefs. Water, with crude *fal ammoniac* diffolved therein, is the beft remedy which
Dr. Mapletoft, fometime profeffor of Grefham
College, confeffes he knows: but, though efficacious, is far from being infallible.

O   The

The milky juice of great celendine, fpurge, pifs-a-bed, or tithymal, will generally take them away.

They are fometimes extirpated, by ufing no other remedy than patches covered with the plaifter of diapalma, or diachylon, with the gums.

The leaves of campanula bruifed, and rubbed upon the warts, three or four times, will generally deflroy them, without leaving the leaft mark behind.

'Divide a red onion, and rub the warts well with it,

The leaves of rue, bruifed in water, with pepper and nitre.

The milky juice of the herb mercury will gradually wafte them away.

The milky juice of green figs, with gum elemi diffolved in vinegar.

From above forty prefcriptions, we have felected the few foregoing, as the leaft hurtful, yet what may be efficacious : the application of cauftics, fuch as precipitated mercury, antimonial butter, and all the acid fpirits, will certainly do much more mifchief than fervice, unlefs you take particular care to guard the parts about the wart from their action by fome defenfive plaifter, efpecially if fuch warts grow near a nerve or tendon; as there are not wanting examples of inflammations, and even gangrenes having been brought on by fuch inattention. And as they generally difappear as perfons grow up, it would be imprudent to run any rifk for the extirpation of them.

Warts are fometimes occafioned by a particular faultinefs in the blood, and then they fpread not only over the hands, but over the

whole

whole body, often to the fize cf a large pea,
or even larger. Thofe in advanced years, who
feed too much on milk, or foods in which a confiderable quantity of milk is ufed, are moft
fubject to them. In order to remove them, the
diet fhou'd be gradually changed, and the perfon
take a pill compofed of the following materials.

Take fix drams of Caftile foap, one dram
and a half of the extract of dandelion, half a
dram of gum ammoniacum ; mix the whole with
fyrup of maiden-hair, and make the mafs into pills
of three grains each, one of which muft be taken
every morning and evening.

It is a miftaken notion that wens are of the fame
nature with warts, for wens are never to be cured
without cutting off, which can only be done
by a very fkilful furgeon.

Corns, a moft vexatious complaint, are commonly occafioned by wearing fhoes too tight, and
made of too tough or coarfe leather : They may
be extirpated by foaking the feet in warm water,
and then cutting the corns gently off with a penknife or razor, always taking care not to proceed fo
far as to wound the foot.

But you will foften the corns, and eafe the feet
more effectually, by ufing a decoction made by
boiling a pound of bran, with a few marfh mallow roots, and two or three handfuls of mallow
leaves, in three quarts of water.

You may apply to the corns a little houfeleek
and ground ivy, dipped in vinegar : even a flice
of frefh lean beef, bound on like a plaifter, and,
renewed as it grows ftale, often takes them away;
a plaifter of galbanum and fal ammoniac, mixed

O 3.   with

with fome faffron, will foften them for cutting away or drawing out ; but, as in the cafe of warts if they rife from the tendons, they can fcarcely be rooted out without danger.

Tight leather fhoes, however, cannot be the only caufe of this excrefcence ; as the ladies are often troubled with them, and their feet are confined in fofter materials. Corns feem rather, therefore, to be produced by friction againft the fhoe ; and certainly do not, like other tumours, arife from any impurity in the blood. The progrefs of corns to their ftate of hardnefs, is very rapid, being generally completed in the fpace of a few days, though the advancement of their growth is more flow. They fhould therefore be attached on their firft appearance, which may be known by the rednefs and pain of the part whence they fpring. When the pain is very violent, the following is a very fuccefsful remedy.

Take equal parts of a roafted onion, and foft foap; beat them up together, and apply them in a linen rag by way of a poultice.

This application will inftantaneoufly appeafe the pain of a corn ; and is equally proper to mitigate thofe pains which return on a change of weather, as from froft to thaw, or the contrary.

If a total extirpation of the corn is defired, a plaifter of diachylon, with the gums fpread on a linen rag, and kept at the part for a fome time, is of extraordinary efficacy : the plaifter ought to be removed every fecond or third night, that the foot may be bathed in warm water, or the fomentation recommended above, in order to foften the corn, which fhould afterwards be cautioufly pared. By this method, continued a fortnight or three weeks

weeks, many painful corns have been entirely eradicated. The plaifter fhould not be too old, as it lofes much of its good qualities by keeping.

Great care fhould be taken in paring corns to prevent their bleeding; cutting too deep has fometimes been produ ive of fatal confequences, as tedious inflammations, and gangrenes, fubjecting the patient to a long ufe of remedies, the neceffity of cutting off a toe, and even to death itfelf.

Callofites or hardneffes, are fometimes found in the palms of the hand, occafioned by handling hard fubftances; often by playing at cricket, tennis, &c. which generally go off of themfelves. They fhould by no means be cut with a razor or penknife, as that only caufes them to grow ftronger, till at length they become as hard as horn itfelf. If very troublefome, an emollient plaifter may be applied to them.

Trembling of the hands is an affliction, or a deformity by no means unfrequent. In the one fex it is often caufed by excefs of various kinds, efpecially in too frequently facrificing to Venus or Bacchus; in the o her by drinking too great quantities of hot diluting liquors; and in both it may arife from having, in infancy, been overdofed with mercurial and draftic purges, either to cure or to preferve h m from worms, fcurvy, &c. and too much bl eding, either for real or imaginary caufes. Sudden frights are of very pernic ous tendency; and may even produce worfe effects than the trembling here fpoken of, the epilepfy being often the confequence of them.

From whatever caufe it originates, much benefit may be expected from the following fomentation.

Take

Take of ſtrong tent wine one quart, red roſes
one handful ; pomegranate rind, two ounces ;
and that of quinces, an ounce ; let them boil
about two minutes, then ſet the decoction to cool,
and ſtrain it through a linen cloth : ſoke the hards
in it when it becomes luke-warm ; heat it again,
and rub the arm from the wriſt to the ſhoulder,
as alſo the nape of the neck, and down the
back

Beating children when at ſchool, eſpecially
upon the hand, is ſufficient to bring on this trembling ; and though not productive of that effect,
ſcarce ever fails to weaken the hands, and render
them leſs nimble for writing or drawing.

When the hands are covered with the ring-
worm, or any tetterous eruption, after taking a
doſe or two of ſome cooling purge, the juice of
chervil may be adminiſtered, to the quantity of a
ſmall wine glaſs full every morning, an hour be-
fo breakfaſt : and as the chervil operates by
peſpiration, care muſt be taken not to catch
cold.

The juice of chervil, is prepared by bruiſing a
bundle of the herb in a marble mortar, and when
well pounded, preſs it ſtrongly through a linen
cloth into a clean earthen or glaſs veſſel, and keep
it in a cool place.

After uſing this juice for two or three days, the
eruption may likely break out more numerous
than before, but will ſoon after gradually
decay.

It is very dangrous to apply hot fomentations
in this eruption; and much more ſo to repel it with
cooling ointment : if the ſkin in an part gangrenes, it may be fomented with a decoction of
bitter

bitter herbs, mixed with camphorated spirits of
wine ; and afterwards a poultice of oatmeal boiled
in strong beer, is to be laid on warm, and renewed
as often as necessary.

It is much better in all eruptions of this kind
to encourage it to come forth as long as the patient can bear the uneasiness, than either to repel,
or carry it off by other outlets ; for all these sorts
of vicious humours (which break out as a kind of
crisis in a disorder,) how much soever they may
be diminished, yet they are rarely evacuated out
of the body, with relief to the patient, by any
other passages than those pointed out by nature.

When the eruption is quite gone, it will be
necessary to purge in the same manner as at the
beginning.

Many people have their hands so very moist,
that whatever they touch retains marks of the
sweat upon it.—Repellent medicines ought by all
means to be avoided ; and the only plan to be
pursued is, to throw it upon the feet; which may
be done thus :

Take some of the oldest green cerecloth you
can procure (not less than two years old) which
cut into soles, and apply to your feet, observing
to wear them both day and night ; this may be
done by sleeping in thin or gauze worsted stockings ;
only every evening and morning observe to wipe
the soles of your feet as well as the plaister with a
linen cloth. Continue wearing them till they lose
their power, which will not be less than ten or
twelve days, when you must have fresh ones. In
a few months the sweating of the hands will be
sensibly abated ; and after six or eight months
is generally cured.

The

The cerecloth has another advantage in removing all callofites and hardneffes of the feet, preferving them foft and pliable; and has the particular quality of rendering them warm in winter, and cool in fummer. Nor does it, when of proper age, adhere to the foot.

Supernumerary fingers and toes are no uncommon deformity. If the fupernumerary part be only a flefhy exuberance, it may be be taken off by a filken ligature tied about the roots, and ftraightened every day, till the part withers and drops off of its own accord. But if the part is bony, it requires the affiftance of a furgeon to amputate it ; though it is perhaps better to leave it unmolefted.

Among many perfons mentioned in hiftory to have had fupernumerary fingers, we may inftance *Anna Bullen*, who had fix on her right hand : as another blemifh, one of her upper front teeth was very mifhapen, and fhe had a tumour in her throat, which fhe partly concealed by her handkerchief : though notwithftanding thefe little blemifhes, fhe poffeffed very extraordinary perfonal charms, and her addrefs and manner were irrefiftable.

Chilblains render the hands exceffive ugly, by the fwellings, and fometimes the chops they occafion. They are caufed by a ftoppage of the tranfpiration in very cold weather, generally in fevere frofts attended with fnow. The beft preventative is to guard againft colds, wearing foft leather gloves, and never foaking the hands in any thing hot.

If prevention is unfuccefsful, and chilblains appear, you may diffolve half a dram of aloes, and

a dram

a dram of camphire in fix ounces of good brandy: dip a linen cloth in this liquor, and apply it to the chilblains, having firft rubbed them gently with the oil of eggs, and continue this till the complaint is removed.

There being no room to doubt but that cold is the caufe of chilblains, it follows that the cure muft chiefly confift in reftoring the blood to its former fluidity and free circulation as foon as poffible. In the internal treatment, on the firft appearance of the inflammation, great fervice may be had from a few glaffes of hot wine, wherein fome cinnamon and fugar have been diffolved ; giving alternately with the wine a fmall quantity of fome fweating mixture: or good ale, boiled with cinnamon, cloves, and fugar, will do as well as wine. It muft be continued fo as to keep the fweat for an hour or upwards, according to the degree of the complaint. And however flight the diforder, this method, is much more certain than, and preferable to any other.

If the perfon is fubject to an annual return of this complaint, the beft prefervative is to anoint the parts affected with petrioleum, or oil of terpentine, before and after the feverity of the winter: when the diforder has fhewn itfelf, the application recommended above may be had recourfe to ; or the afflicted part may be wrapped in a fwine's bladder dipped in the laft mentioned oil ; taking care to avoid cold by proper clothing.

The itch is doubtlefs more properly a difeafe than a deformity, yet when it appears upon the hands and arms, efpecially of women, it is certainly one of the moft difguftful fpecies of the latter that can be prefented to the fight. It is fufficiently well known to render defcription unnecefiary.

One

One of the moſt certain internal medicines is the Æthiops mineral, which may ſafely be relied upon.

For external uſe, take a quarter of a pound of ſulphur in rolls, and holding it with a pair of tongs, ſet it on fire, letting it drop into an earthen veſſel containing a quart of white wine : putting the wine into a bottle for the following uſe.

Pour as much of this wine into a baſon, as is ſufficient to waſh the hands, and let them ſoak in it for a quarter of an hour. This muſt be renewed ſeveral times a day, taking care that the ſame wine is not uſed twice.

This is indiſputably a moſt *elegant* remedy, and at the ſame time is equally, if not *more effectual*, than all or any of the ointments now in uſe for this complaint ; the moſt part of which are overloaded with mercury, and have often fatal conſequences.

Even when thoſe critical eruptions (which appear about the end of ſome diſorders, and prognoſticate a cure) continue too long, and threaten to deform the ſkin, this lotion may be ſafely had recourſe to, not being in the leaſt of a repellent nature. Beſides, that this ſulphurated wine renders the hands ſoft, ſmooth, and white.

The nails are the principal organ of touch, and makes one of the greateſt beauties of the hand, when opened : they ſhould be pretty long, of a lively colour, with a white creſcent, or ſemi-circular ſpeck at the root : the root and ſides ſhould enchaſe themſelves inperceptibly, and as it were loſe themſelves in the ſmall fleſhy border which ſurrounds them. This border ought to be ſmooth and without breaks.

The

A material use of the nails is to strengthen
the ends of the fingers and toes, and to hinder
them from being inverted towards the convex side
of the hand or foot, when we handle or press
upon any thing hard ; so that they serve rather
for buttresses than shields. The extremity of the
nail does not adhere to any thing, and grows as
often as it is cut. The colour is owing to the
vessels underneath the nail, the body of which is
transparent, and exhibits a lively red in a state of
health. It is proverbially said of men of great
courage, that they have blood in their nails;" the
roseate hue of which is generally an indication of
a lively courageous temperament ; and whenever
the blood ceases to flow, the nails becomes pale,
and of an ashen colour.

The Romans had their nails cut by artists, who
made a profession of it.

The Chinese pique themselves on their excessive
length : and among them, indeed, it is a charac-
teristic of rank and quality ; as those who follow
any manual employment cannot preserve their
nails in the same manner. The ladies usually
wear a thin case of gold upon the extremity of
their nails, to preserve them from accidental
injury.

The nails are often bare at the roots in such a
manner, that their joining is quite exposed, like
a picture that is not joined to its frame : for the
roots and sides of each nail should be chased into
the flesh round about as into a frame, and this
ought to be so exact as to come to a level with
the nail by means of a small pellicle that comes
little forward upon the nail in the form of
crescent.   T

To preferve the nails in a ftate of elegance, you muft take care never to foak the fingers either in oily or acid liquors; refigning them to the operation of that natural balfam which nourifhes them, and by the means of which thefe borders increafe and are renewed.

That blacknefs which fometimes gathers between the flefh and the top of tho nail, may be removed by bruifing two or three four grapes, and rubbing the juice upon the part.

The nails are often rendered crooked by ufing a tooth pick, pin, or ear-pick, to take away the dirt that gathers between the extremity of the nail and flefh, which makes the extremity feperate from it, and affume a hook-like form.

When they are allowed to grow too long, the nails are very ugly ; but you fhould take care, in cutting them, not to make them too fhort. Their edges fhould never be cut down below the ends of the fingers, nor fhould they be fuffered to grow longer than the fingers. When the nails are cut down to the quick, it looks as if the perfon were a mechanic, or a fidler, to whom long nails would be troublefome ; and if they are longer than the finger ends, and encircled with a black rim, they feem as if he were engaged in fome dirty laborious employment.

When the nails are accuftomed to be kept very fhort, the flefh at the top of the fingers is apt to rife above them in the form of a pad, which becomes an exerefcence, and a real deformity; befides being always accompanied with dirt entangled about it, which fticks fo clofe that there is no wafhing it away. It is a deformity not eafily to be corrected, on account of the pain which the nail occafions when growing, by pufhing againft
the

the flesh which overgrows it, and compelling you to cut the nail when it becomes of that length, and thus the deformity continues.

The nails, from a superfluity of nutriment, may become too large and thick. To remedy this, scrape them gently, but pretty often, with a bit of glafs, or a very sharp knife, taking care not to go too deep, for fear of hurting the membrane which lines the infide of the nail, and which abounds with tendinous fibres, extremely fufceptible of pain: or you may apply an aftringent plaifter of the following ingredients.

Take equal parts of maftick, lapis calaminaris, bole armoniac, roots of biftort, angelica, and tormertil, reduce them to a fine powder, and with a fufficient quantity of rofin, wax, and turpentine, make it into a plaifter, to be applied over the nail, and continued feveral weeks, only renewing it occafionally.

To promote the Growth and Regeneration of Nails.

Take two drams of orpiment; manna, aloes, and frankincenfe, each one dram; with fix drams of white wax; make them into a liniment, which apply to the part with a thumb-ftall.

To remove Spots from the Nails.

Incorporate together, over a gentle fire, one dram of myrrh, with two of Venice turpentine; fpread a plaifter of this upon a piece of fine filk, and apply it to the nails, when it will foon remove the blemifh.

Or, With half an ounce of bruifed flax feed, mix two drams of white wax, and an ounce of honey; make them into a thick ointment, and apply as above.

P   When

When nails become black, in confequence of a bruife, or other accident, you may apply a plaifter made with capon's greafe, and oil of chamomile, each one dram; flower of fulphur, two fcruples; powder of cummin feed, ten grains; oil of rofes, a fcruple; incorporate them into a plaifter with a fufficient quantity of diachylon.

Whitloes, or felons, an external diforder that affects the finger, and generally is the occafion of the nail coming off, is much more dangerous than ufually imagined. It is an inflammation at the end of the finger, and often happens in confequence of a bruife, a fting, or a bite, and fometimes is the effect of corrupted humours in the internal parts of the body: though moft common to the ends of the fingers, yet it often affects other parts of the body; however the nature of the malady is always the fame, and requires the fame fort of remedies.

The firft fymptoms of this complaint are flow, heavy pains, without heat, rednefs or fwelling; but foon afterwards, the heat becomes intolerable, the part affected becomes large, and the fingers next adjoining fwell exceedingly. Sometimes the whole arm is inflamed, and the pain is fo violent, that the patient is deprived of fleep. When the diforder arifes to fuch a height, the patient, as in all cafes of inflammation, muft be put upon a regular, cooling diet.

In order to procure a difcharge of the corrupted matter, the part affected fhould be dipped in water as hot as the patient can bear; but when the pain becomes extremely fevere, a decoction may ufed made of mallow flowers, boiled in milk mixed with a little bread; and if a few white lily

roots

roots and fome honey, be added, it will be better. When there is a neceffity for making an incifion, in order to let out the putrid matter, the part muft be dreffed with following plaifter.

Take half a pound of red lead, one pound of oil of olives, and four ounces of vinegar, boil them together till they are reduced to the confiftence of a plaifter, then diffolve in the liquid mafs one ounce and a half of white wax, with two drams of camphire, ftirring the whole together till they are properly mixed.

Or, Take pellitory of the well, cut as fmall as poffible, and mix with it a proportionable quantity of hog's lard; wrap it up in feveral papers, one over the other, and place it in afhes, fufficiently hot to reaft the pellitory of the wall, and incorporate it thoroughly with the lard; fpread this liniment on a piece of brown paper, wrap it round the whitloe, and apply a frefh dreffing at leaft twice a day : and that it may give the fpeedier relief, fpread the ointment thick.

We are not born with any greater propenfity to make ufe of one hand than the other ; and this neutrality is preferved after birth ; fo that if a child is not accuftomed to employ the right hand oftener than the left, he will either be *ambi-dexter,* which is rather an advantage than a defect; or left-handed, which is one. Parents fhould take care that their children employ the right hand in preference to the left, in prefenting and receiving any thing, becaufe politenefs has made it a cuftom: but where is the inconveniency of opening a door, cutting a bit of bread, or holding a glafs of liquor with the left hand?—or is it not rather an advan-

tage?

tage? An inability to use the left hand is very
strongly felt, when there happens a wound of
the right; which would be obviated by accustoming ourselves to use both equally.

The thighs and legs are often rendered crooked by
suffering children to walk before these parts have
acquired sufficient strength to support their body,
in which case you will observe a child to prop his
knees one against the other to support himself;
you must thereupon prevent him from walking
any more, and make him sit as much as you can,
till his legs become stronger; otherwise they will
immediately begin to grow crooked, and become
so deformed, as to render assistance unavailable.

On the first discovery of any tendency towards
crookedness, a small plate of iron may be applied
upon the hollow side of the leg, and fastened with
a linen roller, which must be made tighter every
day till it sufficiently compresses the part that projects; and that this pressure may not hurt it, you
must put a large compress under the bandage, on
that part of the leg. The iron should not be
applied upon the bare skin, but let there be some
folds of linen cloth put between them. If the
child is young, you must by no means apply any oils
or emollient ointments to soften the bones, which
are already too feeble; but if he is grown up, they
may have their use.

From negligence in turning out the toes, or
from affectation in turning them out too much,
the feet contract a deformity, less disagreeable
than many others, yet certainly worth the trouble
of correcting, as it is not only boorish and aukward, but an impediment to walking with facility,
and more so with dignity.

Being

Being early taught to dance is one of the best correctives we can prescribe; together with admonition and reproof on the part of the parent. When the person is grown up, reflection on the deformity, with a sense of pride, will greatly contribute to overcome it.

Very much depends upon the nurse's management with respect to almost every deformity. A strong pressure upon parts so susceptible of impression, and which increase so fast as the members of a child, may produce numberless accidents: diforders in the bowels, obstructions in the glands, and ftrangulation in the veffels, are often the sad effects of this violent compression. How many feeble chefts and weak ftomachs are there, occasioned by the veffels which diftribute their liquors to thofe parts, being deprived of their tone f o n having been too much comprefled. We : re happy to know that the practice of fwathing is greatly upon the decline. Nature fhews her refentment of this practice, by making deformity to be fo often its confequence : Deformity is indeed peculiar to the civilized part of mankind, and is generally the work of our own hands. The fuperior ftrength and agility of favages is entirely the effect of their hardy education, of their living moftly abroad in the open air, and of their bodies and limbs never having fuffered any confinement. —And even when limbs are crooked, bindings, irons, or whatever gives pain, frequently adds to the evil; for the child, to eafe itfelf of the irkfomenefs of fuch applications, often acquires a new twift, and thus brings on an additional deformity; whereas, probably, were it left to nature, the actions of the mufcles, when unreftrained, would

con-

contribute much towards recovering the due formation and ftrength of the limbs.

Children are more particularly liable to fprains, in the purfuit of their diverfions and exercifes, than grown-up perfons, and againft fuch accidents, the greateft caution can be of little avail. Whenever fuch an accident happens, it is advifed by fome to plunge the foot immediately into cold water; which is certainly a treatment that ought to be obferved; for the cold water contracts the ligaments that were too much lengthened by the ftrain which they fuffered, and hinders a fluxion of humours to the part. You may likewife employ the following remedy. Mix the white of an egg with a few drops of the oil of rofes, and a thimbleful of alum powdered; fpread this upon a comprefs, and apply it to the fprained part, faftening it with a bandage, which muft be pretty tight.— Take this off at the end of two days, and the third day foment the part with fome warm wine in which you have diffolved a little falt: and lay on another comprefs dipped in the wine, binding it as before. The fomentation to be repeated every other day till the complaint is removed; after which you may apply to the fprained part an aftringent plaifter, fpread upon a bit of leather, and kept on by a roller.

When the foot has been much fprained, it fometimes happens, that although it is cured, yet the patient ftill feels fomething of the pain whole years afterwards, and cannot walk without uneafinefs all that time, efpecially upon uneven or floping ground. The limb or member where a fprain happens, ought to be very cautioufly exerted till it has attained its proper ftrength.—

The

The limbs are sometimes ftrained in fuch a manner that they afterwards become paralytic.

There is a deformity of the feet called bolt feet, in which they refemble thofe of a horfe : it is very common, nay almoft univerfal among the inhabitants of the iflands in the Black Sea ; which they hide by wearing fhoes of ordinary fhape, but having that part within, which the foot leaves void, filled up with cork, or ftuffed with wool. Whenever this happens, it may be greatly relieved by frequently pulling, but very gently, the toes of the child : and a bandage may be wrapped round each foot, prefling moft upon the fides of it.

A few other defects, which deferve a little attention and correction fhall clofe the fubject.

Some people have a waddling way of walking, which either proceeds from ill habit or weaknefs : the firft may be corrected by care and attention ; the latter may be removed by bathing : wearing girdles fo as to comprefs all round the belly, and be ftrong and well furnifhed towards the haunches; and alfo frequently fomenting the loins with a decoction of red rofes and pomegranate fhell, boiled in ftrong tent wine.

Others acquire an unwieldly aukward way of moving, which proceeds from this, that when we take children abroad to walk with us, we do not proportion our pace well enough to theirs , which, however, is of the greateft confequence. For the child endeavouring to keep up with the perfon he accompanies, ftretches his legs beyond what their fize conveniently permits, and thus accuftoms himfelf to long ftrides, whence he contracts a clownifh habit of walking, that it

is by no means an eaſy matter to break him of ;
without mentioning the injuries it gives birth to ;
as rendering the child aſthmatic, or cauſing ſome
relaxation or perhaps a ruptureof the veſſels in the
thorax.

There are others again who can neither walk,
nor ſtand, nor even ſit with any tolerable grace or
dignity, which is ſufficient to draw upon them
the contempt and ridicule of genteel company. It
is not eaſily conceived how advantageous a graceful carriage and a pleaſing addreſs are upon all
occaſions ; many a ſenſible man has loſt ground
for want of theſe little graces ; and many a one
poſſeſſed of theſe perfections alone, has made his
way through life, who otherwiſe would not have
been noticed.

The dancing-ſchool is the firſt ſtage for the
acquiſition of ſuch lighter accompliſhments, ex-
cluſive of its utility as an exerciſe ; where if a perſon learn to walk well, preſent himſelf well in
company, and move his head and arms gracefully,
it is almoſt all that is neceſſary ; and when joined
with attention to the manners of thoſe who have
ſeen the world, will ſoon make a proper behaviour
habitual and familiar.

H E B E.

B O O K   IV.

On the *Preservation* of HEALTH *and* BEAUTY *in general.*

———————Ye finiling band
Of youths and virgins, who thro' all the maze
Of young defire, with rival fteps pu.fue
This charm ——— Tell me———for you know,
Does BEAUTY ever deign to dwell where HEALTH
And active Ufe aré ftrangers ?———

AKENSIDE.

BEAUTY is a kind of idol, which has had its votaries in every age and climate, its empire is perhaps as antient as any other, and certainly in many refpects much more defpotic. The mifchief with which beauty ftands indicted, fhould not, however, make us forget the real advantages which it procures : as when united with virtue it conftitutes the happinefs of polifhed fociety.— The union is natural, it renders virtue more
charming,

charming, while she irradiates beauty with still fresh graces. They are two sisters, two inseparable companions, designed always to appear together, to set off and recommend each other reciprocally; for, in reality, beauty is the virtue of the body, as virtue is the beauty of the soul.

Before we proceed, we must presume to lay it down as an incontrovertible maxim, that beauty can never exist without perfect health ; a healthful constitution, and temperate habit of body, is the very ground-work of beauty ; and though art may assist in polishing her admirable workmanship, in correcting some accidental blemishes, and acting as the handmaid of nature, yet unless she contributes her force to the preservation of these curious models, these master-pieces of creation, "the porcelain clay of human kind," as Dryden expresses it,—they cannot but sensibly decay, and lose their purpureal lustre.

Female beauty, so far as it respects the face, can have no influence or fixed operation, founded in truth and nature, but two. First, as the complexion or symmetry of features denotes health, and all the other animal qualities, dispositions, and affections, which are generally supposed to be the concomitants of it; secondly, as the countenance, expressions, or formations of the features present or indicate to the observer, that the *mind* or *soul* within this earthly casement strictly corresponds to, or is by nature assimilated with those marks of external beauty.

It is not meant, as a conclusion from these remarks, that every woman who bears about her strong marks of animal health, is therefore an object of love or enjoyment, or that every woman, **who**

who is deemed handfome muſt therefore convey to the beholder an idea of beneficence or innate virtue, as well as of external lovelineſs. And it is even farther allowed, that there are women who, though not within the idea of beauty, or in abfo-lutely perfect health, have yet great power to captivate and purſuade.

Though theſe conceſſions are admitted, and though the *likings* of mankind are as various as their faces, and as different as their ages and con-ditions ; yet this by no means militates againſt the principle here laid down, which however li-able to ſome exceptions, muſt in the *abſtract* command aſſent :—viz. " That a *ſound mind* in a *ſound body* * is the great origin of all love and af-fection."

External beauty denotes health and animal per-fection ; *ſuch* a countenance denotes virtue and goodneſs; but,if between the ſexes no other proof could be adduced, the conſtant toils and aſſiduities of the women demonſtrate it beyond all doubt.

White and *red* are the conſtant concomitants of health in this climate ; where nature has denied them, the ladies are always *ſolicitous* to ſupply that defect; and among *w men of faſhion*, and *women of another claſs*, they are generally ſucceſsful in their endeavours.

Again, all the milder and fotter diſpoſitions, which are infeparable from virtue, are always af-fected or borrowed, where nature has been un-kind. Meekneſs, modeſty, a foft tone of voice, abftemiouſneſs at table, a placid, benign counte-nance, a continual ſmile, a defire,at leaſt an *affec-ted* defire to be pleaſed at *every* thing, gentle man-ners, and all thoſe borrowed mental charms,

which

---

* Mens fanis in corpore fano.

which are too frequently caſt off with the *wedding garments.*

This makes us revert to our firſt principle, and declare, we are clearly of opinion, that the idea of beauty originates in apparent *animal* health, and that of virtue in the joint ſymmetry and *expreſſion* of the *countenance.*

Upon this principle we now proceed to the *ſupplemental* part of this treatiſe, or the means of acquiring and preſerving beauty by *natural* means: for hitherto we have only endeavoured to teach the method of diſguiſing deformity, or palliating defects by the aſſiſtance of art.

The temperature of the *air* has a remarkable influence on the complexion ; ſo much ſo, that a characteriſtic colour marks the bulk of the people of every ſoil ; thoſe who live in temperate climates are generally fair and ruddy, while the nearer we approach the Equator, the colour gradually becomes more tawny, till at laſt it ends in the total blackneſs of the Ethiopian. To preſerve complexional beauty, it is therefore neceſſary to avoid the extremes of too cold or hot an air, the impreſſions of which are very forcible, and very deſtructive.

The effluvia from marſhy lands, ſtagnant waters and other noiſome exhalations, affect a delicate complexion almoſt as much as they do delicate lungs ; the bleak coldneſs of a north wind, evening dews, fogs and miſt, are all deſtructive of nature's lillies and roſes. Too dry and parching a wind wrinkles and chops the ſkin ; while the bleak and piercing air makes it rough, contracts the pores, and hinders that kindly tranſpiration,

piration which is fo conducive to health, by carrying off the fuperfluities of humours, arfd fo favourable to beauty, by giving foftnefs and luftre to the fkin.

As a friend to that fex on whom we depend for all the focial happinefs of life, it behoves us to mention every circumftance which experience evinces to be ufeful for the prefervation of health; and fcarce any article is more effential than *Cleanlinefs*. Many of the diforders among the lower claffes of people are owing to a neglect in this po.nt; and many confequences of the moft difagreeable nature refult from fuch a habit. Cleanlinefs is faid to be the fofter-mother of Love; beauty indeed, moft commonly produces that paffion, but cleanlinefs preferves it;

'Tis Beauty points, but Neatnefs guides the dart.

Of all the nations in Europe, the Englifh females are acknowledged to poffefs the pre-eminence in beauty and chaftity, though they are as generally marked for a neglect of thofe arts which are fo neceffary to heighten the former, give delicacy to the latter, and add poignancy to the pleafures of love; *agrémens* in which the French ladies are thought much to excel.—The ufe of the *bidette* is fcarcely known in Britain.

It is, indeed, among the dregs of the people only that the difagreeable nuifances alluded to, are generally to be found; but there certainly exift many degrees of deviation from perfect cleanlinefs, which if not fenfibly injurious to health, are extremely offenfive to delicacy. Nothing fullies beauty fo much as this kind of neg-

Q ligence,

ligence, as on the contrary nothing fets it off to fuch advantage as cleanlinefs. There is a power in it which irrefiftibly attracts the affection, and for which no other perfonal endowment can compenfate; and an indolent difpofition is the general companion of inattention to this article. As perfpiration is much the fame over the whole furface of the human body, there can be no reafon affigned, why the other parts fhould not be more frequenty wafhed, and general bathing more univerfally practifed. This is certainly the cuftom in the eaftern countries where the ladies are the moft tenacious of preferving their beauty; and of which Lady Montague has left fo full an account in her letters. Warm baths are indeed generally had recourfe to, and therefore cannot be fo injurious to beauty, as is fometimes reprefented, or the force of cuftom muft be wonderful indeed :--this happy confequence refults from them that diforders of the breaft are very rare among thefe people.

Pure water is indeed the grand cofmetic of nature: others may eventually injure or difguife the complexion, but water alone is that which makes it fhine with genuine luftre, gives beauty and effulgence that no compofition can beftow, and, like the ftreams which endowed with immortality, protracts the duration of health.

Cofmetics, however, on many occafions, may properly and innocently enough be had recourfe to; and among a variety of *natural* ones which may be ufed with fafety and advantage, bathing. or wafhing with *milk*, efpecially that of goats or affes, has been much recommended for rendering
the

the fkin fmooth, delicate, and giving it a polifhed glofs. The Roman ladies were particularly attached to this cuftom, which is ftill much practifed in the eaftern countries. The juice of the *birch-tree* is juftly celebrated for giving a beautiful, bloom to the complexion; as is alfo pimpernel water, which we have already mentioned.

Though we have already given a choice of very elegant and artificial preparations, yet we cannot well omit the celebrated *Queen of Hungary's Water*; the annexed account of, and recipe for preparing which, were found in a book of devotion belonging to her ferene Highnefs, Donna Ifabella, dated the 12th of October, 1652;—

"I, Donna Ifabella, Queen of Hungary, aged feventy-two years, and being very much indifpofed, was cured by the following recipe, which I had from a hermit, whom I never faw before nor after. By the ufe of it, I entirely recovered my ftrength. It may be ufeful to others. The king of Poland propofed to marry me; which I refufed, for the love of God, and the angel from whom I had this recipe.

" Take what quantity you pleafe of the flowers of rofemary; put them into a glafs retort, and pour in as much fpirit of wine as the flowers can imbibe. Lute the retort well, and let the flowers macerate for fix days; then diftil in a fand heat."

This well-known water is ufed by way of embrocation, to bathe the face, when diluted with common or with rofe-water, and often alone to the limbs, or any part affected with pains or debility. Two tea-fpoons full, in a glafs of rofe,

Q 2   hyfteric,

hyſteric, penny-royal, or briony-water, may be taken two or three times a week, in a morning faſting, and will diſpel gloomineſs, brace up the nerves, and invigorate the whole ſyſtem: but muſt be always uſed cold, whether taken inwardly as a medicine, or applied externally.

It muſt be obſerved, that there is a material difference in the qualities of the ſimple and compound liquids for waſhing the face; the want of attention to which has introduced a prepoſterous practice in coſmetics.

Nothing for inſtance is more common than to recommend Hungary-water, and milk, indiſcriminately; yet 'tis very evident from the nature of theſe lotions, that they act in a manner directly oppoſite to each other, and muſt accordingly produce very different effects. Milk is endowed with a ſoftening, relaxing quality, and may be of very great advantage where the ſkin is rough and dry, and has ſuffered from the injuries either of extreme hot or cold air; whereas, on the contrary, Hungary-water, and all others of a ſpirituous compoſition, are of a hardening and aſtringent quality, and muſt actually prove detrimental in ſuch circumſtances as require applications of the oppoſite kind.

In order, then, to form a judgement when milk and the cooling lotions on one hand, or thoſe of the ſpirituous kind on the other, are moſt proper for beautifying the complexion, let it be laid down as a general rule, that wherever the ſkin is ſmooth and ſoft, the blemiſhes of the face will be beſt removed, and the complexion preſerved cleareſt, by the moderate uſe of the hotter kind of waters;

but where the skin is rough and dry, milk, and the oily preparations (page 80) will be most successful.

Another rule, by which we may pretty justly determine the preference of these applications, is, by considering the particular constitution of the person, to which the texture of the skin is generally correspondent. Thus a youthful vigorous person will reap greater benefit from the softening than the spirituous washes; while the contrary will be the effect in one of an opposite constitution. Those of a blooming complexion will also generally be more injured by hot than cooling lotions; though the case will be different with people who are pale.

But to determine the matter with still more certainty, if the face is moist, and sweats in the morning, or, if after washing it with water, the towel with which it is rubbed, appears more than ordinarily foul, it may be concluded that the skin is of a relaxed texture; and that consequently the spiritous or astringent applications will be more proper than those which are softening.—At first, it will be necessary to be cautious in the use of the former, and to dilute them by the addition of a little water, that they may not stop the perspiration, and thereby not only injure the complexion, but produce more fatal consequences.

Indeed, whether recourse is had to the softening or spirituous washes, the use of them ought to be continued no longer than till the state of the skin is rectified, for otherwise the opposite extremes might be incurred. On this account, it would be proper to discontinue the use of them for a few

days,

ſays, now and then, in order to obſerve what effect
has been produced : if the conſtitution of the ſkin
appear altered, they ought entirely to be laid aſide,
or only uſed ſparingly, and on particular occaſions.

If *Exerciſe* be conducive to health or beauty, it
will not be difficult to account for the preſent de-
generacy of conſtitution in the female world,
owing to an almoſt entire negligence in that article. A country life has always been ſtrongly
inſiſted upon as conducive ; but whether the activity of life, and ſimplicity of diet which is uſually
practiſed there, may not be of as much conſequence as the change of air, admits of enquiry :
for little of that weakneſs exiſts among people
whom faſhion has not yet corrupted, or whoſe
fortunes do not enable them to enter into the
modes of diſſipation. Whatever effects, however,
may reſult from the diverſity of a town or country
life, there is certainly an infinite difference in
point of health between a life of activity and indolence. A very ſlight review of a faſhionable
town-life would ſhew how far it is conſiſtent with
health as depending on exerciſe.

Ten in the morning is an early hour to find a
lady of faſhion riſen from her ſlumbers ; three
hours are perhaps little enough to allow for breakfaſt and dreſſing, when the exerciſe of twenty
minutes or half an hour, by way of airing in a
carriage, is thought a ſufficient waſte of time from
the agreeable chit-chat of the drawing-room.
Convivial entertainments ſucceed, which generally laſt till it is time to attend the opera, the
theatre, or a card-party ; ſo that the only degree

of

of exercife experienced from dinner till the hour of retiring to reft, confifts in the jolting of a carriage through half a dozen ftreets, or a few agitations of the arm, by dealings a pack of cards.

If this ftatement be juft, what muft be thought of the tendency of a life of polite diffipation? Scarce more than half an hour in the day is employed in any kind of profitable exercife.

Of all fedentary amufements, the opera and the theatres may certainly be indulged with the leaft injury to health. The greateft inconveniences are the clofenefs and heat of the place, a circumftance often prejudicial to delicate conftitutions. But the paffions excited in thofe places are of the more generous kind, and united with fentiment, confpire to improve and polifh the attentive auditor: no fordid motives appear to influence the mind, or tranfport with that violence obfervable in gaming —As the paffions to which theatrical entertainments and gaming give birth, are totally oppofite on their nature, fo likewife is their influence on the features; to which the former give the moft agreeable caft, and fhew a abfolutely neceffary to a total conqueft of the heart.

Among the exercifes which a town life admits of, dancing is one of the moft elegant, and moft conducive to health ; it keeps the body erect, puts every joint and mufcle into action, brifkens the circulation of the blood, renders the mind chearful, adds grace and vigour to the whole frame, and above every other exercife, fets off beauty to advantage.

To

Too great indulgence in *Sleep* is as injurious to beauty on one hand, as exceffive watching is on the other. The former renders the body dull, heavy, and lifelefs, while the complexion becomes difcoloured and the face looks bloated : wakefulnefs and anxiety exhauft the fpirits, dry the moifture of the body, and hardly leave blood to crimfon the cheeks with a vermillion blufh.

Temperance, and a choice of food, have a controuling power over the features of a lovely face ; and the fair-one who wifhes to preferve her charms, fhould not be too much addicted to the ftudy of kitchen-philofophy. Ceres and Bacchus may be excellent companions, but too clofe a connection with them will be deftructive of beauty.

The *Paffions* only remain to be confidered, in regard to their effects on health and beauty : nothing has a greater influence on the lovelinefs of the human frame than thofe violent agitations of the mind which frequently attend the ill-fuccefs of a gaming-table.—*Quadrille* will murder beauty. —Were thofe effects as lafting as the paffions are intenfe, it would indeed be fatal for the power of female charms.

Fear and *Anger*, as tranfitory emotions, have likewife but a tranfitory effect, though too often indulged, prove prejudicial to beauty : the ebullitions of anger procure a temporary relief and gratification ; and the apprehenfions of fear are difperfed by removing of the object that caufed it. The effects of *Grief* are much more fatal, and acquire ftrength from duration; its impreffions are made more lafting by reflection, and the means generally employed to turn its edge, anfwer little other

other purpofe, than to convert it into fixed melancholy—the wretched harbinger of the whole
train of nervous diforders; and too often of the
confummate of human misfortune, the deprivation
of thofe faculties, which diftinguifh the human
race among the works of the Deity.

How a paffion fo amiable and engaging as that
of *Love* can be conceived to effect the health, is a
problem more eafily folved by inftance than argument; daily example furnifhes us with innu-
merable proofs of the faireft ftructures of health,
and the moft vigorous conftitutions being overturn-
ed by an excefs of the moft pardonable weaknefs
that can actuate the human breaft.

Congenial fouls take fire at the pure lamp of
love, without regard to rank, fortune, or circumftance, and burn during the exiftence of the vital
fpark; nor is the flame to be extinguifhed by the
mandates of authority, the interference of advice,
or the letter of the law. Indeed, the moment any
paffion becomes calm enough to liften to the dic-
tates of reafon, advice ceafes to be neceffary.

From the difappointment of this paffion, fpring
corroding care, oppreffive melancholy, unavail-
ing complaint, and all the health impairing attendants of hopelefs love; and hence, alfo, lofs
of appetite, difturbed reft, hypochondriac diforders, and too often confumptions, to end the fad
cataftrophe.

We have, therefore, to obviate as much as poffible the fatal effects of difappointed paffion, when
followed by bodily diforder, and to prevent female delicacy from being hurt by divulging the
complaint,

complaint, added a concise selection of medical advice from the most eminent of the faculty, carefully divested of whatever might offend the ear of chastity.

One of the usual consequences of refusing love the sacrifice that he demands, is that complaint which is known by the appellation of the *green-sickness*. It is attended with a viscidity of all the juices, a sallow, pale, or greenish colour of the face, a difficulty of breathing, sickness at the stomach, dislike of proper food, and an unnatural desire of feeding on such things as are accounted hurtful, and unfit for nourishment. The thighs, feet, and parts about the ancles, swell and pit towards night; there is an universal dulness and disinclination to exercise; and any brisk motion, is attended with difficulty of breathing.

When the disorder proceeds from a disappointment of the connubial engagement, or a settled inclination after marriage, the health and happiness of the afflicted patient should supersede every consideration of rank or fortune in the party, where no moral causes intervene. But if matrimony be judged improper, then recourse must be had to physical remedy.

In a constitution inclining to the *em bon point* or jolly, and where the veins are well stored with blood, bleeding will be highly proper to begin the cure, and to be succeeded (especially if the evacuations that are naturally expected at this period seem any way obstructed) by the following medicines.

Take Ruffi's pills, fifteen grains,
  Salt of steel, five grains,
  Oil of savin, one drop:

           Make

Make three pills, for a dofe, which fhould be taken at going to bed, drinking after them a glafs of white wine, and continuing the fame courfe for ten or twelve days.

Or the following tincture may be fubftituted in the room of pills, where they happen to be difagreeable.

Take Tincture of Hiera, half an ounce ;
    Compound fpirit of lavender, and
    Tincture of caftor, each half a dram.

Mix for a fingle dofe.

Thefe medicines, however, muft be continued for ten or twelve days ; taking frequently a glafs of penny-royal or briony water. And after ufing either the pills or the tincture for that time, recourfe may be had efpecially, in delicate habits of body, to the following electuary.

Take conferve of Roman wormwood, and damafk rofes, each one ounce and an half.
    Salt of fteel, two drams,
    Saffron, half a dram,
    Powder of cardamons, one fcruple,
    Syrup of rhubarb, a fufficient quantity to
    . make an eluctuary.

Of this, about the quantity of a large nutmeg may be taken twice a-day, obferving to ufe exercife. But to women of a robuft and fanguine conftitution, Dr. Mead has greatly recommended from two drams to half an ounce of *Tincture of Black Hellebore*, to be taken three or four times a-day.—The good fenfe of every prudent mother will
be

be able to make the neceffary diftinctions in regard of conftitution.

To forward a cure, the lady fhould be placed in a pure air, drink tea, barley-water, and other attenuating liquors, warm, and made agreeable to the palate ; the food fhould be nourifhing ; but light, and moderate exercife will be highly ferviceable, notwithftanding the difficulty and uncafinefs that attends it, and the great antipathy of the patient to any kind of motion.

Sleep fhould be moderate, and taken at a due diftance from meals ; and every attempt fhould be made to keep the mind from anxiety, by procuring and fuggefting a continued change of amufement.

When this diforder appears at fo early a period, that it cannot properly be attributed to any defires or inclination that might bring it on, or before Nature denotes, a change in the conftitution, the following electuary may be prepared, and made ufe of without a doubt of its efficacy.

Take Steel filings, half an ounce,
Species of diambræ, two drams,
Conferve of Roman wormwood, fix drams.
Oil of cinnamon, three drops,
Syrup of faffron, enough to make an electuary.

Take the quantity of a nutmeg twice a day, drinking after it a glafs of hyfteric or penny-royal water.

In very obftinate cafes, the cold bath, with the mineral waters of the Spa, are efficacious : or an infufion may be made in lime-water, with chips of guaicaum, faffafras, and faunders, a little Gentian and Cngelica-root, winter bark, and Roman

man wormwood, with the addition of fteel filings ;
'this may be drank inftead of the Chalybeate waters, and will frequently anfwer the fame purpofe.

There is ftill another enemy more dreadfully
fatal to female charms than any yet enumerated,
and from which worfe confequences are to be apprehended, as the caufe is more likely to be concealed ; and even-the difcovery would tend rather
to excite reproach than pity, as the parties, by a
criminal indulgence to their own inordinate paffions, have been *folely* inftrumental in caufing the
complaint. Too many of the fair fex, efpecially
in their younger years, have frequently fuffered
from fecret attempts to procure to themfelves thofe
delights, which Heaven has intended only as the
effects of the moft holy and legal union. It is
with no little pain we venture to animadvert upon
a fubject, the bare idea of which muft caufe a
blufh in the face of delicate fenfibility, and it
would be a happy circumftance for themfelves, if
their fenfe of virtue were equal to their fenfe of
fhame, and precluded any neceffity for admonifh-
ing them againft the vice, or giving them any precepts to remedy its confequences.

The immorality of fuch a conduct needs no
reprobation, nor is there any human law to deter
its practice : nor; indeed, need there be any other
punifhment than felf-confcioufnefs !—but without
expatiating on the heinoufnefs of the offence, we
fhall only point out its fatal effects upon the conftitution :—here it relaxes the whole frame, brings
on a variety of difeafes and inconveniences, caufes hyfterical diforders, and by draining away the
radical moifture, occafions confumption ; ruins

R   the

the complexion, makes it pale, fwarthy, and haggard, and is the total deftruction of *beauty*. And what effect the confideration of this mult have upon the fpirits of any woman who finds herfelf in thefe deplorable circumftances, and reflects that her misfortune is owing to her own fault,—it will not be difficult to conceive.

When fufficient refolution can be fummoned to quit the practice of the guilty pleafures, before the conftitution is radically injured, and there are few cafes fo bad but may be relieved, let them adhere to an unremitting courfe of the following prefcriptions, which are moft peculiarly adapted to reftore their decayed tone and vigour ; though the effects are fo many and various, it is difficult to give one prefcription that will anfwer all the various intentions of cure.

Take Biftort roots, bruifed, one ounce,
    Roots of Cyperus and Galangal, both
      bruifed, each two ounces,
    Roots of Ofmund royal, cut fmall, two
      ounces,
    Ifinglafs, cut fmall three ounces,
    Archange flowers, and red rofe leaves,
      three or four handfuls each.

Boil them all in two gallons of water, till it comes to fix quarts, and then ftrain it off —A quart of this decoction may be drank every day ;—half a pint in the morning, a pint after dinner, and half a pint at night; but in neither cafe not immediately after taking medicines.

Very great attention fhould be paid to diet, which fhould confift of milk, eggs, jellies, light broths, and every thing of a nutritive kind. The *beef tea* is a pleafant and proper liquor.

The

The white of a new laid egg, well beatten together may be deluted with half a pint of milk, feaſoned with ſpice, and ſweetened to the taſte. — Panadas, prepared from biſcut, &c. with ſugar, and Rheniſh wine, or lemon or orange, are agreeable. Fiſh, particularly, ſhell-fiſh, chocolate, ſago, occaſionally with a glaſs of good generous wine, will be highly beneficial. The Peruvian bark will prove eſpecially ſerviceable, accompanied with the uſe of the Bath, Briſtol, Spaw waters, and moderate exerciſe.

To a ſtrict adherence to the foregoing advice, the following medicine may be added, which is admirable adapted for reſtoring the tone of the veſſels, and re-eſtabliſhing a good texture of the blood.

Take of compound powder of arum root, half
    a dram and candid nutmegs, two ſcru-
    ples.
Angelica and orange-peel, candied, each
    a dram, prepared ſteel, three drams.
Conſerve of garden ſcurvy-graſs, and con-
    ſerve of Roman wormwood, each three
    drams.
Compound powder of roſemary flowers,
    half an ounce.
Syrup of candied ginger, enough to make
    electuary.

The quantity of a nutmeg may be taken every morning faſting, and about four or five hours before going to bed at night, drinking a glaſs of bitter wine after each doſe. A fortnight or three weeks continuance in this courſe is generally attended with the happieſt effects.

For

For external application, a decoction may be made of gall-nuts with red wine, and a few cloves, into which dip a linen compress, and apply it to the part.—

Or the following injection (advised by Dr. H. Smith) may be equally useful.

Diffolve half a scruple of Roman or blue vitriol in two ounces of spring water, and inject a small quantity every night at going to bed.

An attention to these medicines, and a virtuous resolve (which will increase with health and strength) to abandon gratifications attended with shame and destruction, may be relied on for answering the patients highest expectations, without hurting natural delicacy by a communication of their unhappy state.

INDEX

INDEX.

Liniments

INDEX.

Sweaty

I N D E X.

F   I   N   I   S.